CW01645976

NOW is NEW

KATHERINE CHIDIAC

NOW IS NEW

STOP STRUGGLING. START LIVING.

By Katherine Chidiac

Published by We Are Loved Ltd

www.nowisnew.co.uk

Set in 8.5pt/14pt Libre Baskerville
Cover / Typeset by © Katherine Chidiac
ISBN 978-1-3999-2335-4

First edition
Produced in London. United Kingdom. 2022.

For ALL our beautiful and creative children.

May you live and share the love.

YOUR FREE ONLINE WORKBOOK!

As an addition to this book, I have created a workbook that you can download and use.

To access the workbook, open your browser and enter

www.nowisnew.co.uk/workbook

#nowisnew

What lies behind you and what lies in front of you,
pales in comparison to what lies inside of you.

Ralph Waldo Emerson

CONTENTS

INTRODUCTION

> No valid plans for the future can be made by those who have no capacity for living now.
>
> Alan Watts

We are probably similar, you and I. We tend to want to be somewhere we are not. For most of us, there is a compelling and imaginary life waiting, where we are finally secure and content. Where we are happily doing all the cool, exciting stuff we would like to be doing. It's so tantalisingly close, but have you noticed it never quite feels like we are there yet?

I struggled for many years. I didn't like feeling bad, so I searched for solutions in the world. I made unhealthy and healthy choices to feel better temporarily. When nothing really worked, this led to more insecure feelings of failure and anxiety. Everyone else seemed to know what they were doing, so I was playing catch up. I began to imagine that I needed to be someone who didn't look like me, who had things I didn't have and did things I wasn't doing. Then I would feel better. I was always busy yet also weirdly stuck. I could not understand why life often felt so damn hard.

Like me, you have probably done your absolute best to do and achieve MORE.

If I could just get this... Just have that... Just do this next thing... Then life will be all good. THEN I can relax.

There is lots of great advice to help us *do* life better. And yes, it may be helpful to create routines, work smarter, meditate, exercise, eat well, enjoy less screen time, sleep better, etcetera. I'm sure you have tried some of these things. But if you are tired of struggling to 'be better' and you are as fed up with being fed up as I was, then you are in a great position: you know what it is not to feel ok—AND you know you don't have to feel that way. You have hope. That is your wisdom, leading you here to the answers you have been looking for. I will show you it CAN be another way.

This is a book about how we are perfectly positioned to overcome our struggles and thrive. Unlike many other methods, the goal is to take stuff OFF our minds, not add more things we 'should' be doing to the mental party.

We will get to the root of what stops us lovely human beings from fulfilling our potential and enjoying ourselves. I'm pretty sure it's the elusive secret of life. **Simply put, we are only ever up against one thing, and it is hidden right before our very eyes... Our own minds.**

Understanding how our beautiful, creative minds work will help us in every area, especially where we struggle. Unfortunately, we are not taught about our minds in school; this most precious resource we use all day, every day, every second we are alive. Yet everything we need or want is found in the perfect system that generates our psychological experience.

When we come to appreciate the genius within us, we realise we get to create anything we want in life. We begin to look in the mirror, into our infinite irises, honouring and respecting the person we see because there is so much more to us than meets the eye.

Miracles do happen within us and all around us, all the time. But we tend to overlook them and focus on what's wrong and where life doesn't feel good. It does not need to be that way. So, let's get ourselves back on track, skipping down the yellow brick road of life and creating wonderful miracles. **But first, are you open to a simple miracle?**

What would be a miracle?

We create space for something new to flow in by asking ourselves questions. You have picked up this book and started to read it; try to get a sense of what you would love to have. Is there one thing you would like clarity on or to change? We don't need to know 'how' it will happen yet; this is an invitation to dream big. What would be a miracle for you?

Allow yourself to get curious and open to the possibility that making miraculous changes might even be quite simple! After all, if now is always and magically new, then we don't know what will happen in 5 minutes, let alone five years. Right now, is the only place we can step out of our current ideas of what is possible into the unknown and create something new. When we settle down and discover the magic of getting present to this precious moment, we won't need to worry about the past or future. We are ok, just as we are.

Life is short, so ideally, it would be less of a struggle and way more fun. Let's go on a ride and untangle you from the things holding you back. Free you up to fly by the seat of your pants. No, not tomorrow, later, next week, or in the new year. Starting wherever you are, here and now. Let's understand what is getting in the way of you living a life you love. What exactly are you up against in life?

What Would be a Miracle?

1.

WHAT ARE YOU UP AGAINST?

> Once we accept our limits,
> we go beyond them.
>
> Albert Einstein

There are not many human beings who glide through life without struggling. Every day is yet another story of someone we perceive 'has it all' struggling in private. It seems that no matter what we achieve, we never live the dream for very long. And we all dream. We have a sense that we too, are capable of doing or having brilliant things.

But here and now is the life many of us are actually living... As we struggle to get out of bed, leave the house and get to work on time. Struggle just to crack a smile.

We may feel like giving up, pulling the sheets back over our heads. *What's the bloody point?* Many of us can barely cope with keeping it together in our own lives. To put a roof over our heads and food on the table feels difficult. Let alone find the resources to help others or, God forbid, face even more problems in life.

But we get up—day after day—dutifully trying to get 'there' to this mythical place where all is finally well.

We may have developed ways of coping with life that perhaps we wish we hadn't, like endlessly spending hours scrolling and refreshing our screens. We work or play too hard, don't sleep enough and become reliant on food, drugs, drinking too much or smoking. Maybe we are trying to control our relationships with other people, money or our bodies. Perhaps we get into the same old frustrating predicaments or arguments over and over again.

Whatever you may be up against in life, be it mental, emotional or physical, your 'struggle' will describe an experience of difficulty and the effort to resist or overcome it. Hope for something better is built in.

Your personal experience

So, my friend, let's get some clarity. Take a minute to reflect and write down what you are up against in life. What is it you are struggling with?

I struggle with ______________________________

Maybe you said something like this >>>

Perhaps you feel clear on why you are struggling. Perhaps not. There may be multiple reasons or just one, but there is some idea that something *must* or *needs* to change for us to be ok.

What are you up against?

Abuse
Addiction
Ageing
Anxiety
Bad behaviour
Being myself
Being busy
Body issues
Bosses or teachers
Choices
Confidence
Death
Decisions
Demons
Depression
Diagnosis
Difficult people
Eating disorders
Energy
Environmental concerns
Exams
Expectations
Failing
Family
Finding meaning
Friends
Future circumstances
Gaining weight
Gender
Getting out of bed
Habits
Having purpose
Health concerns
Identity
Job / Career
Lack of opportunity
Lack of confidence
Looks
Losing weight
Loss
Loneliness
Mental health
Money
Motivation
Not being good enough
Other people
Overwhelm
Overthinking
Parents
Parenting
Passing exams
Past circumstances
Politics
Pornography
Pressure
Relationships
Religion
Repetitive thinking
Results
Self-harm
Selfish behaviour
Sex
Sexuality
Sleep
The state of the world
Telling the truth
Uncertainty
Work

Page for Reflection

On a bad day, we look out at the world and try to judge how we are doing compared to others—in our work, achievements, finances, families, relationships, fitness or appearance. *I should be doing better,* we think. Life is not working out how we expected. We can easily get down, lose confidence and motivation. We may switch off, retreat and withdraw from others, bury our heads in the sand or quit. This can leave us feeling depressed and even hopeless.

We feel stuck. Stuck not doing what we would like or stuck repetitively trying to do more. Out of anxiety, we tend to overdo things. We go at life hard, but we may become hectic, manic and prone to mistakes. We slip into hyper mode, bouncing all over the place, reactively doing lots but often getting absolutely nowhere.

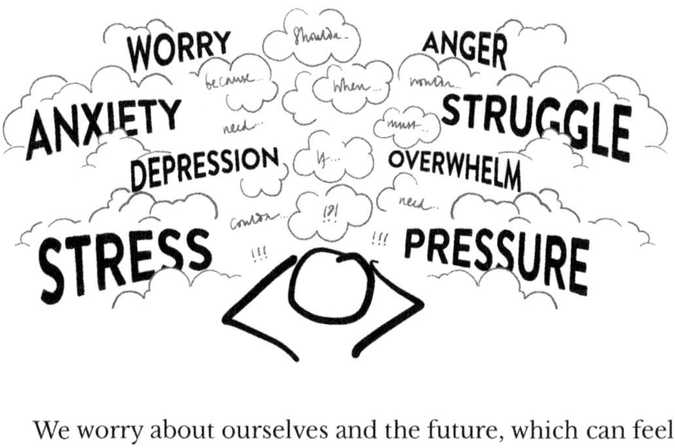

We worry about ourselves and the future, which can feel stressful and overwhelming. We become exhausted from thinking, planning and trying to be positive.

When life feels like this, the little things often push us over the edge. We struggle to control ourselves and may be prone to losing it. We become angry or abusive at minor infractions, constantly getting into arguments—even harming ourselves or others. If this is us, we probably blame and resent others for our problems.

Maybe we feel unlucky, even singled out, cursed or somehow destined to suffer. *Why me! Why does this always happen to me!? It's not fair!* Or we blame ourselves entirely, developing a deep, gnawing insecurity that is bound to haunt everything we do. *What is wrong with me? I am just so useless.*

So, whilst what we struggle with may differ, thankfully, there are common signposts to where life is not feeling easy. Recognising them will become extremely helpful to us in creating a life we love.

What do you notice is happening for you? I would like you to choose one or two things we identified earlier that you struggle with and would like more clarity on. What are some of the feelings you experience?

When I struggle with ____________ I feel ____________

Maybe you feel something like this >>>

Once you have written out a few examples on a page, read aloud what you have written.

Are you enjoying your life when you experience these feelings? Do you feel confident, motivated or empowered? Do you feel able to take your next steps to change freely? Probably not. This is often your reality, and it sucks. It is just not that helpful to spend our lives feeling bad. When we don't feel ok, life feels serious and complicated.

What are you up against?

Aggressive	Hopeless	Rejected
Angry	Hurt	Resentful
Anxious	Indecisive	Rushed
Bored	In denial	Sad
Close-minded	Infuriated	Scared
Compulsive	Insecure	Shut-down
Confused	Impatient	Shy
Damaged	Irresponsible	Stressed
Depressed	Jealous	Stuck
Desperate	Judgemental	Tired
Disappointed	Lonely	Untrusting
Disconnected	Lost	Untrustworthy
Disrespected	Messy	Unclear
Doubtful	Mistrustful	Uncomfortable
Down	Needy	Unconfident
Drained	Negative	Unhappy
Embarrassed	Out of control	Unmotivated
Energyless	Overwhelmed	Unstable
Exhausted	Panicked	Unsupported
Fearful	Perfectionist	Unworthy
Fed up	Powerless	Useless
Frustrated	Pressured	Victimised
Furious	Regretful	Worried

We just want to feel better.

Feeling like a failure is tiring. We are banging our heads against a wall, and we KNOW we don't have to, yet we can't seem to stop. Doing the same things and getting nowhere fast is such a waste of time.

Page for Reflection

I knew I was not doing so great when I texted the guy—again. Like a junkie, *I'll just try him one more time. Maybe he lost his phone?* I couldn't stop myself; I felt compelled to do it. After all, he was the only thing that could make me feel ok again. I totally knew I was off track as I stayed up night after night writing compulsive lists and trying to order my entire life. And I damn well knew I was wildly off track as I sat on the floor of a strange bathroom, having thrown up my dinner. Again.

Sadly, knowing I was off track did not help. I could not stop and did not know how to even begin asking or looking for help. I struggled on, feeling more and more alone, ashamed and useless. I was desperate to sort myself out and fully aware it did not have to be this way. *What's the matter with me? Get it together love.*

So, I'd pick myself up, dust myself down. Go out in the world and look for the highs. Numb the pain. Wake up, not remembering what the hell happened the night before.

But unfortunately, my struggles and suffering didn't seem to go away. No matter what I did or how hard I tried, I eventually ended up on my own, feeling like a failure. I began to hate myself for it. Which led me to make bad choices, and so the cycle continued.

Why do we do such destructive things to ourselves? What would compel us to self-harm, take drugs, medicate or drink ourselves into oblivion? Well, obviously because we cannot bear another moment feeling this crap. We shouldn't have to. We are looking for something—anything—to feel better. We want to feel ok again. Find the flipping off button and relax. Sometimes causing harm is the best we can come up with. It ticks a few boxes because we are not only desperate but angry and frustrated with the world and ourselves.

If we are lucky, our medication of choice will get bad enough that we are forced to seek help. Why do I say lucky? Because many of us can live our entire lives never really enjoying the ride. We hold it together just enough to keep going and not fall apart.

Often, we are advised, 'It's ok not to be ok'. This is true, but it doesn't feel ok at all. We probably don't want a life of accepting the devastating mental health conditions that afflict more and more of us. *Ummmmm... No thanks!* We want to feel good again.

The human race continues with great effort to feel and do better, finding many solutions to this problem. We have developed a myriad of teachings, techniques, mantras, books, advocates, coaches, therapists, counsellors, groups and forums. The thing is, they don't seem to be sustainably working for us.

It's funny because most of us also enjoy the luxury of phones, computers, running water, electricity, dishwashers, washing machines and cars. Clever people are solving all our everyday problems. We have never had so much help.

Now we are not so busy surviving; we have more time to enjoy life, right? But the high levels of anxiety, depression and mental health issues today tell a strange story.

We are struggling more than ever. We are apparently falling apart. Our communities seem to be falling apart. Many of us feel in crisis, drinking from an empty cup with nothing to share. There is something wrong, we know it, and we feel it.

But the problem is not what we think it is. The problem is what we think.

As individuals, we have veered off track in the way we are thinking about ourselves and life. This is totally and utterly innocent because our state of mind is not a personal failing or lack of strength. Our state of mind reflects what we have been taught and come to believe is true.

However bad things may seem, there is always something new to see that will help us. A fresh perspective is available when we head upstream to the root of our problems.

Going upstream

Once upon a time, there was a tranquil, little village on the shores of a vast, sweeping river. A woman was doing her washing on its banks when she heard cries for help. Without thinking, she dived in and pulled the stranger to safety. A few hours later, a fisherman came across another person drowning in the current; he used his rod to pull them ashore. Each day the villagers found more and more people flailing in the water, so the village elders organised them to watch the river in shifts. By the end of the week, the frantic villagers were pulling people from the rushing river every waking minute. They were doing their best, but things only seemed to be getting worse.

Many hard months passed, until one clear and sunny day, the wisest elder in the village announced she was leaving. The other villagers were angry; they begged her to stay. Every spare pair of hands was needed to pull people from the river. They didn't understand how she could leave them amid such a crisis. Nevertheless, they watched her walk away.

Despite their bitter disappointment, the villagers threw themselves back into their work of rescuing people from the river. They went on tirelessly for many weeks, saving as many as possible.

Slowly but surely, it became apparent there were less and less people in need of being rescued. Then came a magical day. The villagers sat in anticipation on the riverbank, but not a single man, woman or child came floating down the river in need of their help. The wise woman returned soon after. Some of the villagers were still angry. They asked her why she had abandoned them to cope with the crisis on their own? She smiled and told them she had gone upstream and taught people how to swim.

As this famous parable so beautifully illustrates, we too are wisely going to uncover the source of our struggles. This is where I finally found my beautiful freedom and peace of mind, and you will too. Because exploring WHY we struggle is how we go from not ok—to ok, how we become secure within ourselves and other people. How we effortlessly take on responsibilities in life yet also create a life of fun and adventure.

So, if you are up for that, the only requirement is to get curious and step out of what we already know. Just for now, and travel together upstream...

2.
GETTING CURIOUS

> We are not afraid of what we think we are afraid of... we are afraid of what we think.
>
> Michael Neill

In my mid-20s, my mum was diagnosed with aggressive cancer and within six horrible months of suffering, she was gone. I was facing the biggest challenge of my life, caring for my mum whilst running a business and looking after a fearless one-year-old boy. I did whatever I could for her, but she suffered a lot and it was hard to witness.

A few days before she died, we moved her from a communal room in the hospice to a small private room. As I set the last of her few treasured items on the table next to her bed, I turned to her and smiled. She stood at the foot of her bed in her nightie and whispered, "they've put me here to die, haven't they?"

I saw absolute terror in my mum's eyes as she said this. I was haunted by this exchange for many years. Why? Because I immediately reassured her. "No mum, you are still doing so well; it will be ok..." *Blah. Blah. Blah.*

I don't even know what I said, but I couldn't meet her there. Not in her terror. I had to make it better. I struggled with this memory for many years. I was full of regrets about my failings; I felt I *should* have done better.

I slept over with her that night, and she seemed fine. I left her the following afternoon, assuring her I would be back first thing in the morning.

When I visited early the following day, she had not come around yet. I slept over again and in the middle of the night, she awoke very distressed. I jumped up in the dark to try and help. She was desperately grabbing at me, trying to tell me something. But she couldn't formulate the words and I couldn't understand her. The nurse ran in and gave her an injection and she immediately slumped. She would never wake again.

Two days later, she was gone. As I drove home from the hospice, I turned up the radio and screamed into the cold night air. I was so angry. Her terror was haunting me. *What was she trying to say? Why had I not helped her more? What the f*** just happened!?*

I experienced the natural grief of losing someone so close. The waves of different emotions depended on how I was thinking about her. Sometimes I would smile as I remembered her tinkling laugh or how she got so excited about the colours in the sky. The way she ran out the room shaking her hands when we watched something scary on her little TV. Sometimes I would feel so sad at her missing out on seeing my son say his first words, starting school or meeting her other grandchildren. Frustrated that after working so hard, she would not retire, relax and do tapestries by the sea.

It is often the things we wish to control that create the most struggle for us. *What if I had got angry with the staff? What if I had stopped them pumping her full of drugs? I should have taken her out of there. I should have taken her home. Should, should, should...*

For years I could not go near that part of London. If I did, I would take the long route so I wouldn't have to go anywhere near the hospice. I was afraid I had failed her there.

But today, I am no longer haunted by what happened. I could drive past the hospice, no problem. I don't struggle with this memory. What happened did not change. The way I thought about it changed. I came to accept and understand that we did the best we could at the time.

Even when tragic and horrible things happen, struggling is not predetermined. Natural feelings of sadness, nostalgia, loss, grief, and fear are inevitable in life and its changing seasons. We move through them. Struggle is not an obligatory part of our adjusting to loss.

We know when we struggle to cope with something because we feel it. There is a need for things to be different from how they are. We have ideas it *should* or *must* be a way that it's not. We don't accept what IS or what might be.

There are so many things I once struggled with that no longer have power over me, even though nothing about the material situation changed. I was stuck there for a while, but I don't feel stuck today.

Can you think of a time you overcame something you had struggled with? Sit back, close your eyes and recall a time you were troubled, upset and did not feel ok. Perhaps it was a particular person or circumstance that challenged you? Something did not go your way; you did not get what you wanted or had an argument.

Page for Reflection

Now reflect on how that same circumstance or person looks today? What has changed?

Isn't it interesting how things don't look the same to us now as they did at the time? How some things that used to bother us don't bother us today. Often the situation supposedly creating our struggle has not changed, but how we think about it has changed.

Our own unique reality

There are many variables in life, and we will each struggle in different ways, with different things, at different times. Some of us struggle some of the time and some of us feel like we are always bloody struggling. There are, of course, those rare and mythical beasts who don't seem to struggle at all.

Why do other people struggle with things we are absolutely fine with? Why do we struggle with things other people don't even think about? There are situations we think we will struggle with, yet we don't. Weird.

We often put these inconsistencies in human experience down to how lucky or privileged we are, genetics, nurture, identity or personality. But is this really how it works?

We think and feel all the time, yet we think about things in our unique way, which forms the entirety of our experience. There is this invisible middleman between the world outside us and our felt reality, our beautiful and creative minds.

Let's explore this by taking an everyday thing many of us will have struggled with at some point—our bank balance—numbers on a screen.

Anything above zero would be pretty impressive to me. I have been in a constant state of overdraft since I was a student twenty-five years ago, no matter how much I have earned. To many people, this balance might be terrifying or shameful; to me, it is perfectly normal.

My wealthiest friend's bank balance would look like bankruptcy and ruin to Jeff Bezos. You see, it's not the bank balance. The meaning and attachments we give these things in our minds create our reality. We often say, *well—it's all relative*, which is true, but relative to what?

What's happening in our life is what's happening. But what's happening is not responsible for putting a feeling inside us. Numbers on a screen cannot create feelings for us; they don't have that power. We will feel whatever we think about the numbers. We only ever feel what we think.

Let's look at another example, our experience of an ordinary spider. Here are my exact thoughts about a spider I found climbing through a mound of washing this morning:

Arghhhhh. Spider! Where's it gone? Hmm, no one here to help me and I have to get this wash on. I have not got time for this!? Oh my God. Where is it? Is it climbing up my sleeve? Maybe it's gone in the machine? I'm not getting it out of there. But it will die if I put on the wash. Ewwww. Dead spider in my sheets? Oh man, I don't want it to die!!!! Sod it. What can I do? Ooooo, [shiver] I hate them.

So, is the spider putting a feeling in me? It sure looked like it, although it's worth considering the spider is there before we become aware of it.

We immediately understand its form when we spy it, judging its size, movement, and proximity. Then, maybe, we consider this hapless spider's implications and future. Or not?

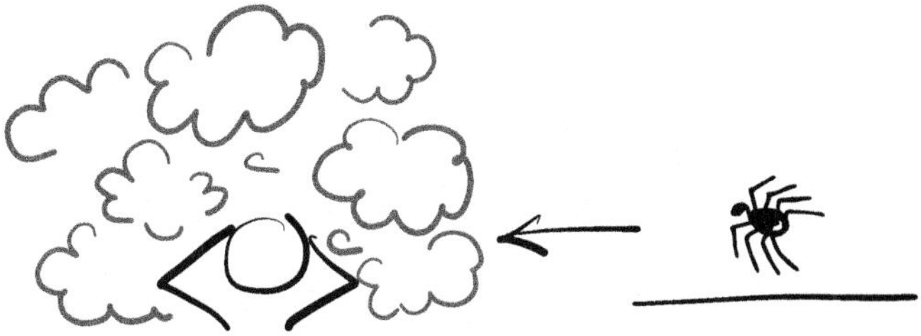

If the spider gave me that experience, then everyone would have the same experience of a spider, right?

Some of you may relate to my pretty pathetic experience of a small creature causing me no actual harm, but many of you will not.

You see for you, it may just be a spider running across the room, but for me, it's my wild imaginings of this creature suddenly running all over me, in my hair, down my top or crawling into my ear to lay eggs. (I know, I was once told this had happened and the idea has terrified me ever since). These vivid thoughts about this rogue spider create more and more fearful feelings as I think them.

It is worth investigating the neutrality of this one fact of a spider—AND our own personal reality, as this will create our reaction. Imagine a spider crossing your path right now. What is your experience?

Like me, many people scream or run in the presence of a spider. Some of us scaredy-cats may elicit spider help, like those kindly souls who will grab a glass and piece of paper and dutifully carry them outside, liberating their little friend. Others will happily kill them. *Where's me flip flop?* Others simply leave them be. And apparently, some people even like them?!

How can a single spider create so many different experiences? It can't. There is a spider, but we will have our unique reality of this spider. This is because our experience does not come from the spider itself but from our thinking.

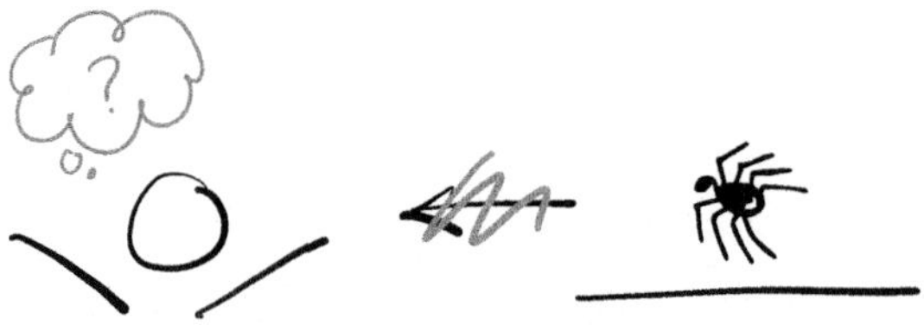

This may sound obvious: we have different ideas and reactions to one thing. I may enjoy the meal, the piece of art, the play, the politician or the preacher... You may not. We know we think differently, yet this fact is often overlooked.

We cannot ever really see things the same. This is the illusion we are all up against. We live in our unique reality of the world; it appears to be the only reality, but it is not real or reality for anyone else in precisely the same way.

The same is true even in our individual experience. On some days, I struggle on my way to drop my kids off at school. I shout at the bumper in front, "Move, you idiot!" and sometimes not. Sometimes I shout at my kids when they endlessly squabble in the car and sometimes, I don't. Sometimes we have a lot of fun. Sometimes none. Same school run, different experience, daily.

It does look like the external changing circumstances create our experience; the car in front, how our family behave, how we look or what work we do. But actually, we can only ever find one reliable variable in our experience, our own thinking, based on what we believe is true about life.

We all just want to be ok.

Life can be a tough gig and we will all suffer challenges at times. How much we struggle with this is a result of how much we accept life on life's terms. But this is not easy to do unless we understand how life works. When we feel bad, there is always an opportunity and invitation for us to get curious. This will create space for something helpful we may have not yet considered. What is going on for us? What do we believe needs to happen for us to be ok?

When we look within, our whole world can change beyond recognition. Think back to all the possible causes of struggle we considered in chapter one. Some of these look like challenges to us, while others seem like no problem at all. You may not worry about losing weight but struggle to gain it, or maybe weight is not an issue? You may not struggle with money, but your partner does. You may feel overwhelmed at work but relaxed at home, or the other way around.

Again, pick one of the things you struggle with. Take some time to explore what belief feels real to you.

I struggle with... *my skin / losing weight / being fit / my partner / friends / money / political ideas / liars etc.*

I struggle with... ______________________

The story we are telling ourselves is that we are not ok unless this changes. So, let's turn it around to reflect this:

I will be ok if... *I have good skin / I am thin / I am fit / I have a great partner / I have lots of good friends / I have more money /*

my political party wins / you don't lie / people are nicer / I am free / I pass the exam / I am successful / the world is ok etc.

Now your turn, jot down one example and then ask yourself the following questions:

I will be ok if... __________________________

- **Do you always feel this?** Is there ever a time this belief does not look true for you?
- **What does this belief do for you?** For example, you may believe *I will be ok if I have more money.* Perhaps you think this will motivate you to make more money? Or maybe you just like terrifying yourself with potential future scenarios?
- **Can you think of someone this belief is not true for?** They don't buy into this idea. Maybe you don't think it's true for them either! They are ok as they are.
- **If you did not have this belief, who would you be?** What experience might become available?
- **And finally, do you feel willing to let this belief of "I am ok if..." go?** Maybe / maybe not.

There is no right or wrong here, but if I were to offer any advice in this book, it would be simply to stay curious. It's fascinating to explore what we think is possible. Because, as

Page for Reflection

Page for Reflection

an adult, we actually make up the rules around here. We get to decide how our lives go. No matter what we have faced in the past or face today, we are only one thought away from all possibilities. This is unbelievably hopeful.

Nothing has been more helpful to me than understanding that we create our experience. *My feelings don't come from what I think they come from—they come from what I think!* It works the same ingenious way for us all. However, the way we think won't change unless we get curious about what we believe.

Beliefs are funny old things. We cannot see them. They don't show up in flashing neon lights indicating they are, in fact, 'a belief'. They are invisible to us. Hidden. They simply look real and we tend not to question them.

Our beautiful minds create our entire and unique reality from these beliefs. The peace of mind and energy we bring to the world are dependent on what ideas we hold about ourselves, other people and the world. They will determine whether we feel ok or not ok in life.

Of course, when we don't understand that our experience is generated within us, we naturally look for the source of our feelings outside of ourselves. This fundamental misunderstanding creates all our insecurity, struggle, and unnecessary suffering. Happily, we can start to uncover the beliefs that may be holding us back today. How do we do this? We can begin to notice where we feel bad.

It is not the fact that we are *rich / poor, winning / losing, fat / thin, fit / unfit, right / wrong or with a great partner...*

What we believe is true about these things will determine whether we feel secure and content in our lives. This is a world of difference.

Life does not happen to us; life happens through us. The implications of seeing through the greatest illusion in life are epic. We finally get to experience everything we ever wanted. But what exactly are we struggling and striving for in life? What do we want?

3.

WHAT DO YOU WANT?

If you don't get what you want, you suffer;
if you get what you don't want, you suffer;
even when you get exactly what you want,
you still suffer because you can't hold on
to it forever. Your mind is your predicament.
It wants to be free of change. Free of pain,
free of the obligations of life and death.
But change is law and no amount of
pretending will alter that reality.

Socrates

A few years ago, I was sitting on my bedroom floor crying. I was trying to get things done but couldn't seem to do anything. I was feeling anxious about a meeting later that day and nothing was making me feel better. Not crying, worrying, list writing or coffee.

Randomly, my best friend Kriss knocked on the door. She lives on the other side of London, so it was rare for her to call in, but she was visiting her brother in the area.

"What's up?" She asked as she saw my swollen face. She did not need to be told; she knew exactly what I was upset about. For several years I had been passionately working on a freelance project that I loved, but I had become increasingly insecure about my role and value within the organisation.

I had been going over and over it, having full-blown conversations with imaginary people in my head for months. My kids quizzically wrinkled their little noses, "mum are you talking to yourself?" *Ummm. Yes I am.* I sheepishly smiled.

I felt desperate for something to shift and to feel ok again. I was constantly trying to work it all out. *Why don't they do something? Why don't they care? How had it come to this? What should I do? What should they do? I need them to do something!*

So here I was bitching to Kriss for the 100th time. She listened for a bit and then asked me the million-dollar question: "What do YOU want, Kat?"

I looked at her blankly. "What do I want?" Erm, that's not what this is about? I haven't got time for this. "Look babe I have a meeting later. I need you to help me work out what I should say. What do you think needs to happen? What do you think they want? What should I do?"

She looked at me firmly and said carefully, "I don't care what they want or need; what do YOU want?"

Errrrrrrrrrrrr...

I had no idea. The long and the short answer. No flipping clue. Bizarrely, I had not thought about that for one single second. I didn't want what was happening. But it was dawning on me, the problem I thought I had may not be the problem at all. *Hmmm.*

That day Kriss lovingly picked me off the floor and dusted me down. She had helpfully got me to the point where I did not spend the whole meeting lost in a sea of victimhood. I still had no clue what I wanted. But there was now a glimmer of hope that perhaps I was not as stuck and helpless as it may have appeared.

I was starting to glimpse the empowering truth. It wasn't my works or employer's job to meet my needs—it was mine. What was it I thought I needed?

This gets to the heart of our struggle. What is lacking for us? What is it we want? No one can know what we want but us. What are we struggling and striving for?

So, if the first step is realising you are struggling, the second step is getting clear today; what do you want? Or, as my friend Thomas, a fantastic therapist and teacher, suggested, I ask more expansively: What would you like?

Being

We all have our own preferences. What are yours? Let your mind wander. Dare to dream. Sit back and get comfortable. Relax and close your eyes. If I had a magic wand and we could create the life of your dreams, what would you like in it?

I want you to get specific. Don't tell me 'lots of money' or 'a nice house'. Imagine the details. We want an exact figure in your savings account. What does your dream house look like? Where is it? What does it have in it?

Is it a new car? If so, what car? What colour, make and model? Picture it, sit at the wheel and cruise in it. If you want a successful career, what type of career? What would success be for you?

You may be looking to have a fantastic relationship. To be a great parent? Auntie or uncle? Godmother or Godfather? How and what does that look like? Is it having more holidays

Have...

and leisure time? Spending quality time with friends and family? Walking on the beach, mountains or in the park more? Getting a dog? Going travelling? Helping others? How and in what way do you want to help others?

You get the idea. Allow your imagination to run riot; what would you like? Paint a picture in your extraordinary mind and write down all the things you would like under the title 'HAVE'.

Now don't get all judgy. Just let whatever floats up be. Don't overthink it; this is not a manifesting exercise. This is a fun way to understand something about the way we work.

Write a story, make a list, do a spider diagram—whatever feels good—but do it. Just right now, as you are, what would you like? Here is mine:

I am in the kitchen of my spacious 1970s house, where massive windows overlook a sandy beach and the shimmering ocean. The wintry sun is shining. The fire crackles, and my coffee pot bubbles away on the large, gleaming stove. I have just done a workout and I feel strong and fit. Here I am, a successful writer who has published many best-selling books. I have hundreds of thousands in the bank I do not need today. I think I will plan a fabulous party for all our friends this weekend. Happy days.

Again, what we would like will not be the same. You will have your own picture of what you would like to have... I have managed to work quite a few of my *I'm sure I would be ok if...'s* in there!

I would be ok if we... *lived by the sea / had more money / were fitter / had more fun :)*

Once you have written out what you would like to have, close your eyes. Let your creative mind go to town again.

This is your reality. Imagine all the details of your life now that you have everything you dream of. Be in it. Shimmy those shoulders and settle in. Waft in the having.

I open the big sliding doors out to the garden on a beautiful clear sunny day. I inhale the sight, sound and smell of the ocean. I can see no mounds of clothes in my kitchen, only a big pot of food on the stove next to a full fridge. My kids are playing cards at the table in front of our fireplace. They are not arguing and moaning. They have not got their heads in a phone or iPad. They are talking and laughing together.

I sigh a contented sigh and mosey into my beautiful wooden study to write at my clean and clear desk. I leisurely open the mail, and my latest bank statement flutters out. There is now a nice long line of numbers (with no minus at the front!). Aaaaaahhhhhhhh. Bliss.

How do I feel in this mini-movie I have just created? Who am I being? Now write the word 'Be' and jot down all the feelings of your dream life. Here is my example.

I am... *Relaxed, present, satisfied, secure, grateful, abundant, free, open, confident, connected, spacious, loving...*

Take a minute and breathe in all these gorgeous words of being. This is what we want. Not the stuff. We just think the stuff will allow us to feel these states of being.

Finally, in our little exercise, I want you to consider: when you are 'being' this being-ness, what do you imagine you will 'do' with your day? When you feel all those lovely words, what do you do?

Would you happily get out of bed, ready to begin another glorious day? Maybe jump in your car and go to the gym? Be more social? Make more time for the people you love?

What do you want?

Be...

Have cool parties? Would you help people around you? Spend more time relaxing doing what you love? Would you still spend all your time worrying, or would you spend time doing exciting new stuff?

I always imagine that when I have what I want and am secure, I will finally live a full life. There is no pressure or stress. I will have the space and presence to do everything I want to do...

Take the dog on long leisurely strolls
Exercise daily
Cook gorgeous fresh food
Take time to relax and just read
Write and create more freely
Make cool jewellery
Confidently share my work with the world
Spend more time being with people I love
Meet new people and go to cool places
Have more fun, entertain and throw parties

Do you imagine it will be easier or harder to get more of what you would like from that kind of being and doing? Yup, I think it will be easier too. It all feels effortless. We are no longer struggling but free to enjoy life. We will be out in the world, doing all the things that enable us to have more of the things we would like.

You see where this is going? That's how we think life works, right? If we have what we want, we will be our best selves and we will do all the things that give us more of what we like. Great! That's a good plan!

Oh, but wait... There's a problem. 99.999999% of the people on this planet do not have the things they 'want' or

What do you want?

Do…

'need' right now. So, if *having = being* and we don't have what we want, how might we feel? It would be easy to be disappointed, defeated, stuck, fed up, pressured, angry, stressed, victimised and insecure. There may be anxiety to *do* and *have* more, and if we can't, we may feel like we have failed. Or that life has failed us.

From this position, where we feel bad about ourselves and life, are we likely to do the things we need to do to have the things we want?

Maybe, but it's pretty hard to crack on with life when we are full of bad feelings. We may oscillate between motivation and apathy. Some days we may not want to get out of bed; we just want to scroll through social media, fill online shopping baskets, watch tv or play computer games. On other days, we are on fire. We get busy walking the walk, somehow finding the determination to persevere and conquer life. Even though we feel a lot of discomfort at times, we push through and drive ourselves forward, not even stopping for a minute to celebrate our wins. We are on the grind. We are in the never-ending loop of doing/having more.

I will be happy or fulfilled when... I will do this because... I need to be able to... I will be ok if...

We think it works as a process. That *being* is a result of *having*. We create a holy trinity of doing, having and being.

DO more >>> HAVE more >>> BE well & happy >>> DO more >>> HAVE more >>> BE well & happy >>> REPEAT...

Take care. This is easy to miss. I have used a fun example by asking what you would like. But there is an innocent dependency we can so easily create. We may not think the new house, flash car or money in the bank will make us happy. For us, it may be our families and loved ones being ok, our health, the state of the planet, changing people's lives and opinions. We get our good feelings from helping others.

We believe we should always do more and work hard—that is what *makes* us ok. Whatever preference or flavour of this misunderstanding we have, there is still a state of being we crave. We *need* something. Fill in the blank.

I will be ok if... ______________________
(*I help others, my family is ok, I am healthy etc.*)

Our being well is conditional on what we *do* and *have*. Me too, by the way. I am writing this wee book right now and can easily fall into a state of fear and pressure. I am dancing around an *I will be ok if...* campfire.

I will be ok if... *I finish this book... I publish the book... people have read my book... people like the book... someone found the book helpful... I have written the next book. HAH.*

It's never bloody ending, right!? Even if we get what we want, we simply move the goalposts.

Our natural capacities

What if I could help you see that we don't need to do or have anything to be ok? That we already have everything we need inside? That we can have all those wonderful feelings we really want at any time:

Security, hope, peace, calmness, contentment, kindness, clarity, wisdom, gratitude, abundance, freedom, resilience, motivation, confidence, presence, love, connection...

Our good feelings are NOT dependent on anything outside of us. These beautiful qualities we crave are generated within us. Fundamental to us all is a limitless capacity for gratitude and hope, even when the world may not appear abundant or hopeful. When bad things happen to our loved ones or us, we can—and we do—deal with it.

Our innate resilient and responsive capabilities are why we are not all sitting in the corner shaking with terror. Because, let's face it, the prognosis of life is not good for any of us. Unfortunately, we will die, as will those we love. Life is brutal like that.

Thankfully we have the internal resources to respond to life as it happens. To get over loss and hurt. We also have an innate proclivity to seek meaning and purpose. To create powerful positive connections—to love and be loved. When we look towards our universal qualities as human beings, we will uncover a reliable source of health—a fountain of life bringing the infinite energy to get up today and go again.

When life looks personal and limited, we have simply overlooked our natural capacity to be ok. We think we are not ok. This innocent misunderstanding is epic. The implications may even be tragic.

We no longer experience and enjoy our beautiful innate states of being. We have become entangled in the dependencies we have created. We are literally bound to struggle. Stuck in wishful thinking and busy minds. So how do we become unstuck and free from struggle? How do we 'be well' more of the time?

4.
BEING... BUSY

Sometimes it seems as if there are more solutions than problems. On closer scrutiny, it turns out that many of today's problems are a result of yesterday's solutions.

Thomas Sowell

So, we come to understand that who we are 'being' is important. This is not a new concept. But of course, we want 'better being'. We want to feel good.

When we experience feelings like stress, worry or anxiety, they are not comfortable and we want them to go away. We are compelled to try and work out a way to feel better and go looking for good feelings.

And because we are such an innovative species, we have got very busy creating 'solutions' to our wellbeing problem. This has perhaps complicated and compounded our 'problems'. We are now not only faced with our deepest insecurities, but a growing and overwhelming list of things we *should or could* be doing to be ok again!? A new never-ending shopping list.

To encourage our wellbeing, we may start following motivational gurus. We take up yoga, exercise, diet, meditate and say affirmations. We post empowering quotes to remind ourselves and help others. We listen to motivating podcasts on mindset and life hacks. We spend a fortune on Amazon and online courses. *This is it! This is finally the thing that will make me feel and do better.*

For many years, I searched for 'better being'. Unfortunately, it was not found in my achievements, popping pills, drinking lots or dancing all night. As fun and fabulous as these things can feel temporarily, they were not the solution. They also seemed to come with some sort of cost or headache afterwards. So, I went looking for my good, healthy feelings elsewhere. I meditated, prayed, chanted, practised, read, talked, listened, tapped... I knew I did not need to struggle with life the way I did.

Maybe I will feel better if... *I practise more/read this book/write more gratitude lists/get into better habits/wake up earlier/create a proper routine/eat better/do yoga/exercise more/meditate daily.* And sometimes this went the way I thought it should—aaaaaand sometimes not.

But what was the hack? I had not found it. The failsafe way to better and reliable wellbeing? To have the energy to be the person I knew I could be. After all, I was searching and practising for a result, right? To 'be better'.

It is powerful when we understand that it is our beliefs and the way we think creating our reality. So, of course, we imagine we have to manage our minds, sort out our thinking or change our beliefs. But here's the thing—that just puts more pressure on us and we can end up feeling worse.

The wonderful states I discovered on the good old journey of life just never lasted. I felt disappointed that all my efforts did not seem to help when I needed them. When I faced a big problem, I was the same as everyone else. All that hard work did not stop me from feeling bad. *Damn it.*

Trying to 'be better' is like doing a 1000 piece puzzle repeatedly but always finding there is a vital missing piece. So unsatisfactory! I rarely felt content and 'happy'. I never felt like the puzzle of life was complete. But I had not understood the simple truth about human beings and life. I had been super busy addressing the wrong problem.

The problem is a perspective

When we pay attention to our good and bad feelings, we see what prevents us from living the life we would like to live.

This is important as what stressed us out yesterday is likely to stress us out today or tomorrow unless we see something new.

When we are dependent on something going our way to feel ok, we are on insecure ground. No wonder we don't feel secure. We can't control life, so we often don't feel we can cope. We live with a whole lot of thinking based on this false premise:

If... __________ (x happens) **then...** __________ (I will be y)

So, for example: *If I win the lottery, then I will be secure / If I get the job, I will feel great / If I can meditate every day, then I can cope / If I forgive my mother, then I will be free / If I don't reconcile my past, then I can't be ok / If I help others then I am good...*

We may believe that if we looked better, had more money and became successful, we would finally be ok, secure and loved. Because if I had my lovely house by the beach, raked in the doh and floated about with my cup of homemade coffee, life would be marvellous. This looks true to us. But it is the root of our problems. We have simply started with the wrong equation.

If x, then y. (Or *x=y)*. Everything following this mistaken idea will inevitably create struggle for us. Why? Because the actual equation is:

If x, then ??? We don't know what will happen in the future, mainly because we don't know what we will think! And what we think will form the entirety of our experience. We may win the lottery *whoo-hooo,* yet develop a whole lot of insecure thinking about needing to give it away, what to do with it and how to keep it. Yup. We are still up at night worrying about money! Nothing has changed.

If we believe there is no choice—**I have to...** *make money / be successful / do more / be more efficient / be free* **to be ok**—we will feel it. How do we feel when we believe there is no choice? *Stuck / confused / overwhelmed / useless / lacking / disappointed / desperate / emotionally unstable / no good.*

After a while, we may no longer believe the life we would like is even possible. We stop believing in ourselves. *Why can't I do this? Why does this always happen to me? Why do I always do this? WHAT IS WRONG WITH ME?*

Helpfully, feeling bad illuminates the hidden beliefs we hold about ourselves and our lives that create our actions or inaction. It is vital to understand this, as there are consequences when we regularly feel bad. We will experience physical effects of mental overwhelm, depression, anxiety, stress, worry, pressure, anger, frustration and insecurity. We embody our emotions. They can physically consume us. We may be not sleeping, feel energyless, lethargic, nauseous or ill. We may find ourselves in physical pain or even severe states of dis-ease.

Thankfully life is full of brilliant humans creating solutions to our actual problems. There are no problems without solutions. But if we don't believe it's possible to move out of the problem, we won't. It's that simple. We have choices. Again, it is not the job of our work, our possessions or other people to meet our needs—it is our job. The circumstance or situation is what it is. It may be a fact that we need more money, but the 'problem' we struggle with is a perspective. This is the game-changer.

We CAN relax, even when we don't know the solution yet. We are ok. We will know what we know when we know it. The answers will become apparent when we settle down into being, here and now, where we are naturally open to new ideas.

Perhaps we will uncover only opportunities rather than problems when we KNOW a different perspective is always available. We have the freedom and potential to replace *I have to...* with *I could...* or *I can...*

I can do more work. I could make more money. Right now, I am ok. And guess what? **When we feel ok, we do ok**.

Finally, a solution...

I became free when I stopped seeking to validate myself by what I do or have. Life became easier when I realised it was not my fault, or anyone else's fault, that I felt bad. It was not because I was useless or wrong either. What a relief! I finally felt relaxed, grateful and fundamentally secure in my life.

Today, instead of thinking my mind works against me when I feel bad, I KNOW my mind is always working FOR me.

This is the elusive missing piece of life's great puzzle. Nothing is broken or missing. Life works perfectly. There is a reason we feel what we feel. It's not random and there is nothing wrong with us. We innocently made up our own equations and rules, then acted as if they were the only reality. We don't need to do that anymore.

The solutions to all our problems were not found in the book, the practice, the meditation, the course, the guru, etcetera. Nothing can give us our ok-ness and all rightness. We were born with it. It is within us before all the trying, aspiring and doing before life gets all personal. Before the illusion that is 'my life'.

> Out beyond ideas of wrongdoing and rightdoing there is a field. I'll meet you there. When the soul lies down in that grass the world is too full to talk about.
>
> Rumi

I did not have to wake up this morning and remember to breathe, blink my eyes or digest my food. Neither did you. We do not consciously heal our cuts, beat our heart or regulate our body temperature. We don't need to grow our babies; they just grow. Nor do we make the trees lush, the sun shine or the stars twinkle.

Even I, the queen of list-making, does not have running my body and making sure the earth spins on my never ending daily to-do lists. There are intricate, interconnected, intelligent systems at play within us and all around us that do the heavy lifting in life. The solar, weather, water and gravitational systems – to name but a few. These complex and interactive systems do not depend on humans. We don't design them or get them right. They were here long before us and will be here long after we are gone. They are present for all of us, all the time.

The more we understand how the natural systems in and around us work, the more we can align with them. We can harness their potential. The more we understand our bodies, the more we can make progress against unnecessary physical suffering. As we have created better optical devices, we have understood the solar system better. We can put satellites into space, fly aeroplanes and call our families across the globe.

It is helpful to know the reliable and universal qualities found within a system that works the same way for us all. Understanding evolves ALL humanity.

This is true for our psychological system, which is always underneath our temporary and personal experience. It creates all thought and feeling and, in turn, our entire reality. Understanding this system IS the health we seek. We are ok—more than ok. We are so impressive.

We don't need to manage our minds or mental health. We are born to perfectly respond to life. I know it does not feel like it at times, especially when we are frightened by our experience, but there is a system that has got our back. Through birth, we were given everything we have ever wanted or needed.

When we start to appreciate how amazing we are, there are vast implications for how we live our lives. It's no longer all on us to get it right. Because we know we are not wrong. We know we are ok.

We stop being so busy trying to get good feelings that are only ever found and generated within us. We can finally relax our shoulders and enjoy the ride. We all have the most precious of gifts...

Our beautiful creative minds.

5.

OUR BEAUTIFUL CREATIVE MINDS

Men go abroad to wonder at the heights of mountains, at the huge waves of the sea, at the long courses of the rivers, at the vast compass of the ocean, at the circular motions of the stars, and they pass by themselves without wondering.

Saint Augustine

There is nowhere better to experience our extraordinary minds than right now. At this exact moment, you must be holding and reading this book? Turning your attention away from the thousands of distractions inside and outside you. Your eyes move 3-5 times per second, scanning and collating complex visual information. You focus on these lines of text, where individual letterforms in black ink create the shape of words you have learned to recognise quickly.

To each of these words, you give meaning in the context of the other words and punctuation marks around them. Within milliseconds you will create a mental picture and understanding of these neutral marks AND decide if you like it.

And it is not just when we are reading. There is this constant transaction happening in our brains. Look up and take in your surroundings. We are actually seeing the light rays reflected off objects that give us the information of form. Our irises widen to allow more light, create depth and perceive colours. Then over 100 million cells send electrical signals to the brain, which turn what you see the right way up! Yeah—apparently, everything we see is initially processed upside down.

All-day, every day, we take in massive amounts of complex sensory data. Our brains interact with what we see, hear, smell, taste and touch to create meaning. We seamlessly form connections, generate pictures and stories, understand and recognise patterns. We analyse and judge all new information against what we already know, deciding its importance and categorising it accordingly.

Our minds intricately interpret the world around us without any conscious effort in every single second we are alive.

The current consensus is that all our thinking originates in the brain: the most significant physical organ and the engine room of our bodies. Thought is often defined as brain activity. That is how it works. Except from what I have gleaned, we still know little about thought and the brain.

Not surprising, given it's said to be the most complex known structure in the universe. I recently read that there are more neurons in our brain than stars in the sky. That's billions with a hundred trillion more electrical connections between these neurons. How magical is that? Our brain is a hive of electrochemical activity sending and receiving information. Hard to imagine the wild electrical dance happening in our heads right now.

We know that the brain is the hub of our nervous system. It processes all our physical and sensory experiences. This is unconscious, i.e. we don't have to do it consciously! Our brains get on with sorting us out silently in the background. As we are busy reading or watching TV, our brains are doing the epic job of understanding all the input whilst still controlling our bodies.

This is busy work. Our brain manages the relationship with other people and the world around us, but it also processes and regulates all our major organs and systems in our bodies, including our respiratory, muscular, skeletal, and neurological systems.

Every second, billions of neurons transmit their electrical impulses throughout our body. Our arm naturally turns the page; our fingers scratch an itch and our body moves to a more comfortable position. We seamlessly respond to barely conscious ideas and suggestions within us.

Without our brains, we would have no experience. A decision may be made to turn off the life-support machine of a coma patient when there is no sign of brain activity. When the brain is dead, we understand there is no life. That vital spark is so evidently gone. The power source is no longer connected.

So, whilst we are still trying to wrap our genius heads around exactly how or why the brain works, we can fully appreciate that it does work. We have this superpower constantly creating our entire reality.

Somewhere in the billions of connections in our brain, we have a thought, which creates a feeling. The electrochemical activity sparked by our thinking instantly transmits sensations throughout our body. This feeling is then further processed and recognised within the brain, creating yet more thinking and feeling. And so it goes around and around over our entire lifetime.

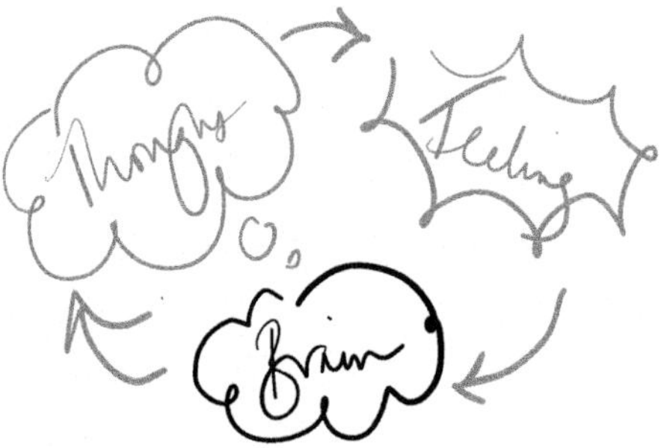

All humans enjoy this innate capacity to think and feel. We experience and feel one thought after another, after another... Our psychological system creates all our physical and sensory experiences. There is an entire formless world we live in that is created in our minds. No one else can see it or experience it; **how we think and feel IS our reality**.

This is the universal way all humans experience life. There is one system AND there is your unique experience of it. Like our experience of the spider, I will feel my thinking and you will feel yours. One thing happening in infinite ways.

The intelligent mind

There is an element of our psychological system that is simply inexplicable. It is currently known by words like 'psyche' and 'mind', which refer to the psychological system's more intangible and invisible components. Here, our experience of life does not appear to be confined to the brain. An intelligent evolutionary phenomenon allows us to generate new connections and ideas. But where do these come from?

It's a bit like knowing our little smartphones are 'smart' because they have a connection. This clever little object is not designed to hold all the information we enjoy from it. *Oh no.* It's not got this infinite knowledge in a teeny tiny hard drive behind the screen.

It is a very clever piece of hardware, but the magic of our smartphones comes alive in the operating software it runs and the connections it facilitates. The hardware has a certain capacity for storage built-in, but it's also connected to the internet or the 'cloud'.

In the ether of our minds, we can find every fantasy and imagining available at any time. When we ask a question, it is entered into a search bar. Instantly the mind and memory are trawled for information and scanned for new ideas. We sit staring off into the distance in our little virtual reality. We can conjure several outcomes to any potential scenario or problem in seconds.

Our mind constantly generates and processes even though we are not conscious of it, even when we are in 'sleep mode'. Our brain is the hardware, with clever, inbuilt software running all the systems to keep the hardware in operation. Then there is its connection to an intelligence that facilitates our infinite capacity to create the new.

But in the context of us, what is this cloud? Is it a collective unconscious? What is the source of this intelligent and responsive electrochemical energy – and where is it from? Somewhere, in the billions of electric dancing nodes within us, is a spark that ignites us. Physicists refer to it as a life 'force', and many others, including biologists, call it 'energy'. Some call it the 'mind', 'source', 'chi', 'higher power' or 'universe', and religions may call it 'God'. I don't mind what it's called. I will call it 'intelligence' in the interest of complete neutrality.

Not our personal intelligence, but a universal intelligence that powers all life.

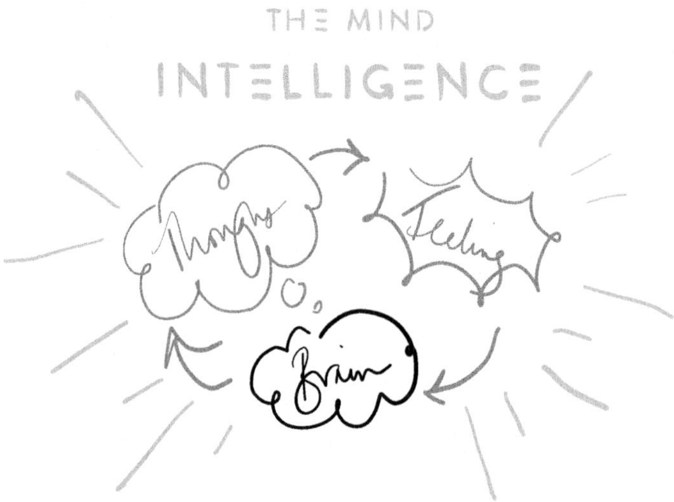

All humans are aware of it. There is a more profound sense of something far greater than our administrative physical and sensory experience. We use the words 'soul', 'spirit' or 'heart' instead of 'head' to describe it.

I have yet to meet a human adult who does not have a concept of some sort of soulful or intuitive state. Perhaps when they listen to music, read, enjoy nature, ponder life or laugh with a small child. When we feel connected, it fortifies us. Here we are humbled and united in our plight of experience with more in common than in difference. We understand that life is not personal but universal. We can appreciate our shared condition and humanity. We recognise our sameness. We value our wonder-full and ingenious psychological system, which brings us a rich and unique experience all day, every day.

Our psychological system only works now.

Luckily, we don't have to live wading through a jumbled mess of everything we have ever seen, thought and done. The brain operates with what we describe as consciousness or awareness. This means we are perfectly built to respond to life and adapt to what is, as it happens.

We experience one thought at a time. What we experience right now IS our entire conscious experience.

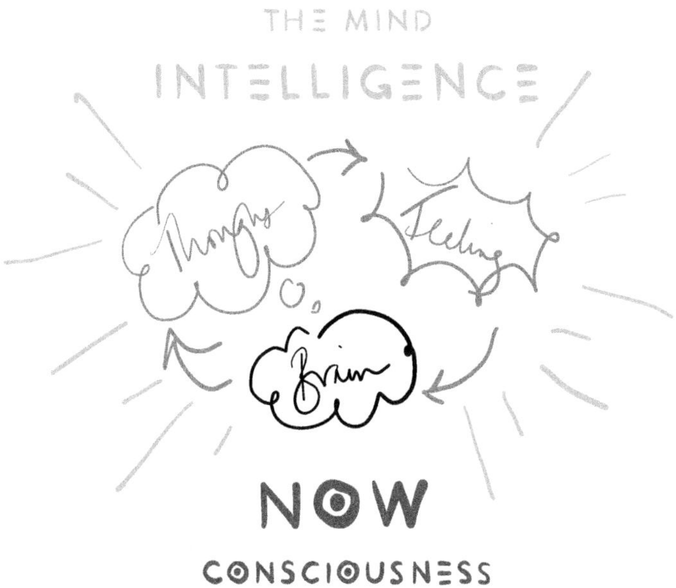

Whether it be experiencing thoughts about the past or ideas of the future—we experience these only now. Our calculations, wildest imaginations and whimsical ponderings also happen now. Whether our experience is good or bad. We feel whatever we think right now. Now. NOW.

Consciousness looks to me to be the energetic ability to form connections and communicate from the smallest cell to the largest solar systems. An inexplicable spark of connection found both externally, with other living forms of consciousness, and internally, within the complex system we call a body. We don't need to DO anything to experience our conscious presence. When we were born, this is what showed up.

This incredible presence is found in us and arguably in all life. It is an innate awareness that is always on and always alert, responsively taking in information or fuel and processing it—ever seeking evolution. This is how we work.

The reason newborn babies are so special is their openness and curiosity; they welcome each new moment. Babies aren't filled with ideas about who they are, what has happened and what needs to happen. They are not full of knowing; they are free to explore and play, to wonder at the world.

So, you may well be sitting there like, *whaaat?* Or you may be like—*yeah, I love this.* You may think this is confusing, complex, boring, kinda interesting, or life-changing. But whatever your conscious experience is, no one else will be having the same one; it is yours exclusively right now.

All the components of our innately healthy minds work beautifully together. If the spark of life is there, then there is the potential to evolve, the capacity to learn and grow.

The brain generates thought and feelings, facilitates consciousness and is powered by the expansive intelligence informing the system. Formless energy constantly and harmoniously creating form within us and all around us.

When we begin to comprehend the creative genius within us, we are no longer tempted to manage it. We see it's bigger than us. Rather we are inspired to not get in its way.

Page for Reflection

6.
BEING WELL

No law or ordinance is mightier than understanding.

Plato

In even our most basic experience, understanding the genius at play is the key to being well. When we uncover the powerful, connecting and intelligent energy within us, we have found the gold at the end of the proverbial rainbow.

We—me and you—don't need to do anything to make ourselves work 'better'. We don't NEED to become more 'conscious', more 'intelligent', or more 'thoughtful'. We are already all these things. We have everything we need built right into the system inside us. There is always the potential for understanding.

We can strive to have all the knowledge in the world, but it won't move or evolve us if we don't understand it. Until we travel upstream to how knowledge is generated and understood, we will be overlooking something vital to make sense of our experience.

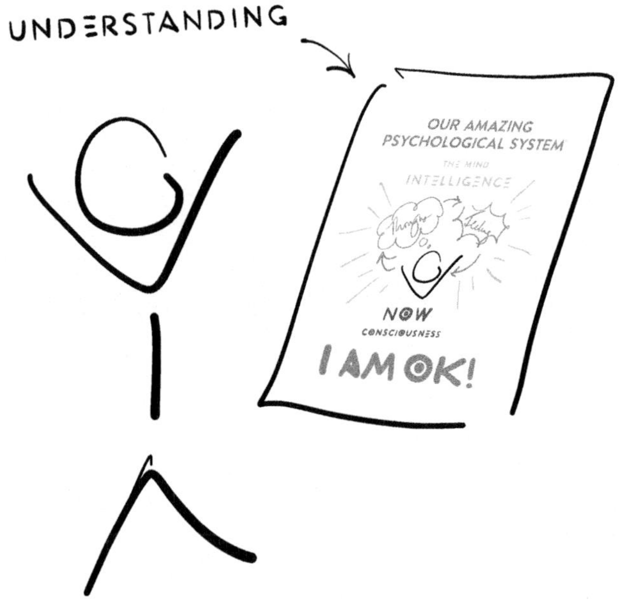

We are bound to struggle to make sense of life if we don't know there is a reliable system creating our reality and how it works. We will feel insecure as we inevitably become fearful and create stress for ourselves.

We look to our experience when we don't feel ok; we need something to happen or change to return to being ok. It does look like that is how it works. We can't see our psychological system. It is invisible to us, so we overlook it and live in the content it creates.

What we *do* and *have* does seem to make us happy, sometimes. How people behave does seem to make us feel good or bad. Our resilience, creativity and intelligence do seem to be personal achievements.

So, of course, when things don't go how we want them to, we are bound to become scared that we can't cope, worried we won't know what to do, insecure we may not get it 'right'.

Why? *Because duh—it is on us to get back to ok? It's our personal strength or weakness, right?* If you believe this to be true, then God help you when life doesn't go your way.

This is THE misunderstanding that prevents us from feeling perfectly equipped to deal with life. We think all good stuff is 'ours' personally. This is what people often call our 'ego', our attachment to it being personal. That all the fantastic things in our lives are down to our hard work and personal intelligence. When we think it's all on us, unfortunately, suffering is in the post.

The good news is that when we understand how impersonal life is, we won't suffer and struggle so much. Because our bad feelings are also not ours personally. It is not our failing or something to feel ashamed of when we are not doing well. We don't need to overcome or better ourselves.

There is intelligence through the system that runs us; our bad feelings are not a sign that something is wrong. Bad feelings awaken us to the misunderstanding at the root of our suffering.

There is a reliable life force bringing us everything we have ever needed. We CAN handle life no matter what we are up against. The world and everyone in it start to make sense. The gifts of life begin to appear all around us.

A deep well of being

We uncover a deep well of being inside us. This is our default setting. Again, like our smartphone, we can wipe the data and return to 'factory settings'. The phone still has the same functionality, but it's not filled with our personal stuff. There is space inside for new applications and data. Nothing wrong with the personal stuff; I love my apps, messages and pics. But if we are having trouble with our phone, it's good to know we can reset any time.

The same is true for us. Beyond our personal experience is a universal place where we all fundamentally work the same. Intelligent energy created exquisite operating systems throughout the universe. When we realise this infinite resource is within us too, we effortlessly evolve.

This natural state of being is full of creative potential. I love to think of it as a bright, warming sun inside. An infinite life force that restores us. Like the sun in the sky, it is always there, breathing light and energy into all the beautiful systems inside and around us. This intelligent energy is the elusive well of being we are all trying to come home to. When we don't feel it, we go searching for it.

Entrepreneurial folk package up things that may spark or evoke it and sell it back to us. But it is only ever found within us. Right now, beyond the weather of your personal experience, this resource is ever-present.

The place I am pointing to will feel familiar. You will know this place because it is always and has always been inside you. It is not mine or yours, but ours.

This is well-being redefined as simply *being well. Good to go. All good. All right. AOK.*

We don't do it; we are it. We can fall back into it anytime and often in the most unlikely circumstances.

Really—I'm ok.

There was a time when I could no longer look people in the eyes; any human interaction ended in tears for me. I felt broken. I imagined people could see the bloody muscle and bone through my skin on the train to work. I felt raw. Messy. *Am I going crazy!?* I could not pretend to be ok anymore.

I quit my job and tried to work from home, a little one-room studio flat in an attractive but smelly house in Camden Town. I was trying so hard, but somehow, I couldn't keep myself together. It was frightening to feel so out of control.

One month I couldn't pay the rent and so I signed on. The state would now pay my rent and give me some money to live. I wept as they interviewed me. I thought I was letting people down and I was a failure. I had no idea what was happening to me and what would happen. I felt like I was drowning, sinking deeper and deeper. There was no dry land to escape to. Nowhere felt safe.

The woman interviewing me worriedly handed me over to a homeless project. I woke up a bit. *Oh Um. Hold on—I have my little place,* I assured them, now feeling like a drama queen. *I'm not homeless!? I have my family. I'm ok. I'll be fine. It's fine. Really! I'm ok. *Sniff sniff. Hiccup.* The more I protested, the more nuts I appeared.

They persuaded me to at least go and see the room they had allocated to me. I agreed. The moment I walked in, I knew it was for me. It was a small attic room with a small balcony surrounded by trees. Standing in that empty sterile room, I felt like I had come home. Because it wasn't the room. I knew I was where I needed to be. I needed to stop for a while. I felt hope for the first time in many years.

One evening, I was lounging on the old plastic chair on the balcony, wrapped up in my duvet, drinking a cup of tea. I gazed up at the sky and the swallows flying over my head. I felt like the richest person alive.

I will never forget the deep sense of wellbeing I experienced there in that little room. I had let go and in letting go I was not found lacking. In that experience, I found a home inside me. All the feelings I had searched for—security, gratitude, freedom and love. There was nothing I wanted or could think of wanting. I didn't have anything, yet I discovered peace. The world was looking after me in the most unexpected way.

In that year living there, all the things I had wanted but struggled to do now came to me effortlessly, not through pushing myself harder but by relaxing. I got a little job, then two jobs and even started a business. My friend Freda told me they needed someone a couple of evenings at the beauty salon she worked in. Another friend mentioned they needed a receptionist in the yoga studio—where you can do free yoga classes! Then another friend, Alex, asked me to do a design project with them. This led to us founding a successful business together. There was a flow and ease to which my life took shape again.

We don't need to hold it all together anymore. We are already held. When we struggle with life and become afraid, it is compelling to think we need to do more. We must work harder to get out of our situation. It looks that way to all of us, me too.

But what we want in life is not found in this wanting and needing state of being. We are too busy to connect or notice the beautiful details in our lives. To be present in the life we already have.

Amazing things happen when we are present. In my story, I moved forward because I had found an ok-ness within that opened me up. I slowed down to life instead of speeding up. There was space in the 'not knowing', which led to new possibilities I had not considered. I found wellbeing in a situation I imagined would feel precisely the opposite.

How often were you on a beach or somewhere beautiful yet did not feel ok? You finally achieved something you wanted and just felt *meh*.

What about those days when you walk down the street and notice the beautiful flower? You smile at your neighbour and feel full of the joys of spring for no apparent reason?

This is because it's not the beach, the achievement, the street, flower or neighbour. How we feel about these things is based on what we think and what we think is based on what we believe to be true about life.

Let's pause for a moment and reflect. Close your eyes and allow a time to come back to you when you felt a real sense of your ok-ness and wellbeing. Don't judge it and work out if that is the best one. Just go wherever your mind takes you, soak it up, be there and feel it. What is it you are feeling?

Maybe you said something like this... *Looked after / peaceful / relaxed / in flow / connected / loving / kind / responsive / grateful*

Page for Reflection

/ wise / generous / abundant / creative / confident / being myself / motivated / hopeful / content / joyful / unlimited / open / free.

Think back to the exercise where we worked out what we would like and how we thought this would make us feel. I bet some of those feelings are here.

Even if you feel in the darkest of places and crushed by life, you will have known these states. They are available to us at any time. We are only one thought away from them—no matter what terrible or brutal things we may have faced.

In the midst of hate, I found there was,
within me, an invincible love.
In the midst of tears, I found there was,
within me, an invincible smile.
In the midst of chaos, I found there was,
within me, an invincible calm.

I realised, through it all, that...
In the midst of winter, I found there was,
within me, an invincible summer.
And that makes me happy. For it says that no
matter how hard the world pushes against
me, within me, there's something stronger–
something better, pushing right back.

Albert Camus

We are always in a magical transaction with the world around us. Taking in information, creating connections and developing solutions. It is in this capacity for creativity that we find a natural resilience. It is how we have thrived as a species. We are designed to get over things and to have new ideas. We CAN move on from hurt and adversity.

Throughout our human history, great thinkers, creatives and innovators have always pointed us home to the truth which transcends time and culture. Because there is only one way we humans work. We have our unique experiences, but it is generated the same way for us all. Once we connect with this profound resource, it nourishes and restores us. We realise our blessings.

Our psychological system is entirely unaffected by our personal experience. Again, we can draw an analogy from another system we all understand—the weather. Sometimes it's stormy, sometimes cloudy, occasionally blue skies. We know the sun is always shining behind the temporary weather and clouds. In the same way, there is always this bright potential energy behind the brief weather of our minds.

The sun always shines.

Recently I was doing the dishes and burst into tears of gratitude for the flowing water. The warm soapy bubbles cleansing away the dirt. I know; I was confused at myself.

I had been considering what genius humans had made this possible for me. The beautiful minds that designed the sanitation systems crisscrossing London, who maintain and fix them, ensuring there is this endless stream of flowing hot water from my tap. So I can wash up.

Needless to say, I do not feel this way every time I do the dishes. Sometimes feelings of self-pity arise within me as I confront my overflowing kitchen sink after a long day at work. I feel completely fed up as I try to scrub old, dried food off dirty plates and lift gunk from the plughole. *Urgh. Disgusting!*

My feelings reflect my thinking, not the dirty dishes or other people. Gratitude arose within me, from the way I was thinking about the running water, not from the water—the victimised feelings, not from the dirt, but my *thinking* about the dirt.

Our feelings are generated within us and are not dependent on things outside us. Not our situation, circumstances or other people. Feelings of gratitude are natural to us when we don't fill up with thinking about what *should* happen. We become free when we notice what is.

We can only get to neutrality and clarity when we don't take things (like dishes) personally. When we comprehend that life is never actually personal, we uncover our ability to respond and even encourage others to help!

We find freedom from unecessary suffering when we remember that our minds are always free. We can think and feel anything and be ok—no matter the experience. When we understand where our feelings come from we have peace of mind. We recognise that it's not our job to be ok and make others ok. We are ok, and so are they.

We can help one another and point each other home, but there is no burden. Life can become more of a pleasure. Less serious.

We are finally secure because we know there is a vitality in life bringing us what we need. We have not been forsaken but blessed with the wisdom right now to survive and thrive. We can finally be content, grateful for we are intricately connected to something powerful within us, everyone around us and our entire world.

The warm rays of our vital life force and the spark of genius within us are always there, shining out of our innate capacity.

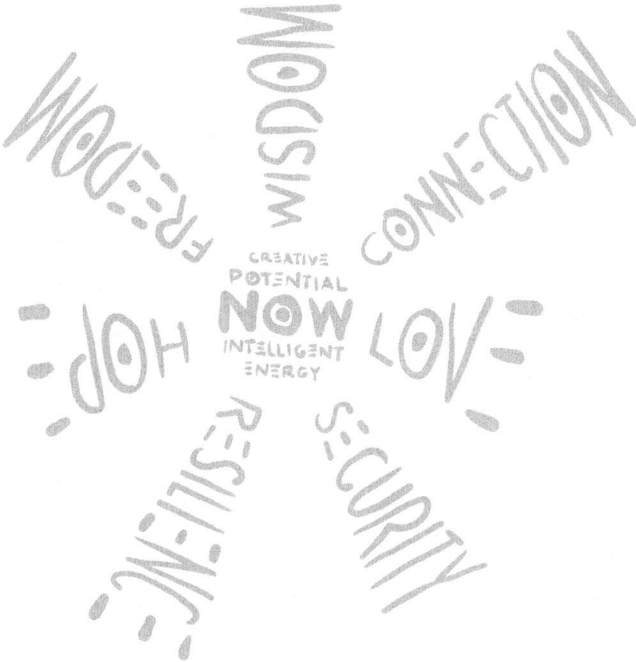

We can remember times of wellbeing and imagine times of wellbeing to come. But we will feel these warm feelings only here, in this precious moment, where life actually happens.

We notice the swallows flying in the sky above us. We see the bees nestling in the flowers. We hear the bird's song. Life comes alive. We notice how others struggle too. We know what is happening for them and we can gently reorientate them back to their innate health and wisdom. Life is simpler than we imagined.

The world feels less scary and more awesome. We have eyes for all the wonder and magic within us and surrounding us.

Does this mean we will be happy all the time? No. It's so unbearably easy to overlook what is right with us and the world and focus on what is wrong.

But this does beg the question—if we are so bloody marvellous, why do we feel so bad? What gets in the way of all this incredible potential?

Page for Reflection

7.
WHAT GETS IN THE WAY?

Knowing how to think empowers you far beyond those who know only what to think.

Neil deGrasse Tyson

Right now, all over the world, other humans are creating all sorts of weird and wonderful new things. But why do so many of us use our gift of creativity to create unnecessary suffering and struggle in our world?

Our lives transform when we begin to appreciate our minds, BUT the minute we look outside ourselves for our feelings, we are in trouble. If we think something or someone can take away our ok-ness and innate freedom, we will—for sure—struggle. There is no choice.

We can find no sun and beautiful blue sky in our experience, only dark clouds and storms. Or worse—endless dull, grey and overcast days. Instead of knowing the sun is still there, behind the clouds, it disappears for us.

Our being ok looks conditional on external factors. This is a terrifyingly insecure place to be.

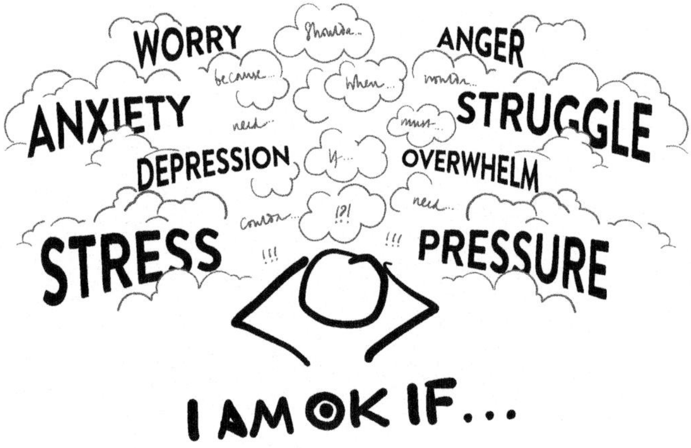

Predictably, we will struggle to find our good and ok feelings again. We feel anxiety and pressure to manage our world. We stress and worry about how this is going and what can go wrong. Eventually, we become overwhelmed, feeling lost and insecure. We look for solid ground somewhere, but where?

Our loved ones? Our job? Our bank accounts? Our bodies? No matter where we turn, these people and things are not reliable sources of good feelings. We have based our ok-ness and security on things that are simply not secure, so we inevitably struggle. We are bound to. We are basing life on a completely illogical and faulty premise.

This would not be the first time we have struggled when we did not understand what was happening in life. Our ancestors were once terrified when the sun disappeared during terrible weather conditions and solar eclipses.

Many ancient cultures worshipped the sun itself as a God. When it disappeared, they believed it was because the Gods were angry with them. They were understandably frightened. They had no means to know or predict what was happening, so they developed prayer rituals or even sacrificed some poor souls to please the Gods.

Clearly, this would not make sense to us today. So, what has changed?

We witness the same phenomenon, a solar eclipse, but we are no longer frightened because we now understand weather patterns and solar eclipses; we predict them, design, and prepare for them. We now know the earth spins around the sun and how the day turns into night.

It seems ridiculous now that people would ever think the sun could disappear.

Many of us have flown in a plane high in the sky, looking down on the clouds below while basking in the sun's glorious rays. We know the sun is still there, no matter the temporary weather.

Well, it works in the same way for our experience. There is a reliable system creating our own temporary and personal reality. It is always 'on', yet it is invisible; we see and feel the unique experience it makes. The experience of horrible and overwhelming feelings we describe as panic, anxiety and depression are scary. We feel insecure.

So, we too developed our own rituals, both healthy and unhealthy. We try everything and anything to feel better. We think it's on us to fix. It's not. Understanding how our psychological system works is vital.

No need to panic

When I was 19, I would get panic attacks. Not all the time, but there was a time when they seemed to get worse and worse. I couldn't catch my breath and I thought I was dying.

It was terrifying because the more I tried to regain control of my breathing, the worse it got.

I told my good friend Lauren, who shared a story of having a severe panic attack in public. A policeman had helped, assuring her she was ok and would be ok. The worst that could happen was that she would faint and her body would resume breathing on its own. It helped her.

When she told me this story, it made sense to me; I could understand it was true. I never had a bad panic attack again. I didn't need to do anything. I simply came to understand something that helped me. The story did not solve the underlying anxiety, but I was no longer terrified I would die. That made a big bloody difference. A whole category of frightening thinking did not occur to me anymore.

So, while I was no longer concerned about my lack of breath, I was still anxious and concerned at feeling so bad. I felt frightened by life and out of my depth.

When someone kindly showed me how my mind worked, like the policeman's explanation, it made sense to me too. I tested it and saw it was true. I now know where true security in life is found. I no longer spend my precious time worrying whether I am mentally ok if I feel extreme emotions. I know these feelings tell me nothing more than how I am thinking. The only thing we are ever really up against. I don't need to try and work out the precise cause of my pain, how to fix myself or the world to be ok.

Realising the sun within us is never gone is a game-changer. We are ok.

Do we understand we have what we need to cope with whatever comes our way right here and now? Are we feeling blessed or stressed?

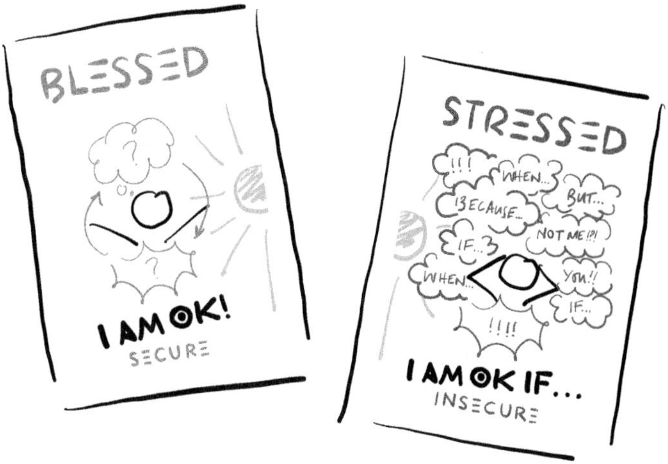

Stressed that we don't have what we need? *I will be ok if...* Or do we know we are blessed with the incredible capacity to be? *I am ok!*

Our experience is NOT random.

There is this pervasive yet unhelpful idea that our experience is random somehow. That quite by chance, we may become mentally unstable and struggle with life. That some of us thrive and some of us don't—just random.

There are theories that it is because of our chemistry, genetics, circumstances, race, gender or culture.

Maybe some of us are just unlucky? Some individuals are just sensitive. Bless them; they find life harder than we do. Some of us are blessed and some are not.

I do not believe anything about our personal experience is random.

Sometimes humans develop beliefs about life that do not serve us. All around us, people seem to be suffering mentally more and more. Literally we cannot do better than we do, when we fundamentally misunderstand how our experience of life works. Our minds will follow a way of thinking that will take us off track. It's a done deal.

When we do not believe we are ok, we start from lack. The way that we think about life is then wholly predictable. If we do not know we have everything we need inside, we will 100% look for it outside of us. Of course we would. When this goes well, we will feel great. And when it does not, we will struggle.

We then see bad feelings as a signal to get super busy—you know—sorting out ourselves, other people or the world we live in.

Perhaps you don't feel great right now? Something is going on that you are struggling with. Something feels wrong. This is the perfect opportunity to get curious.

Let's take a moment or two to reflect. Do we know we have been beautifully designed to cope with whatever we face right now? What have we started to understand about our experience? Does something outside of us look like it can make us feel bad or good?

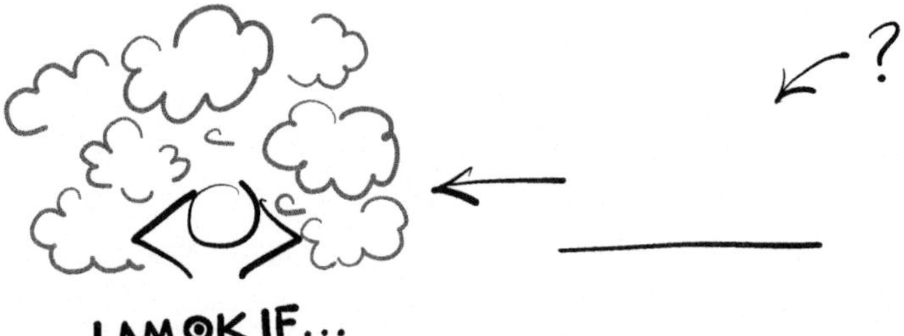

When we find ourselves not feeling good about something, we think it is that thing making us feel bad. We decide it MUST change.

I will be ok if... ____________________

Our minds are bound to fill in the blanks and we will naturally start to think about what *should* or *needs* to happen for us to be ok again.

Again, remember our spider? How we think about it will determine how we feel. It's not the spider or anything else that is the cause of our feelings, however scary or real they feel. We will only feel whatever we think.

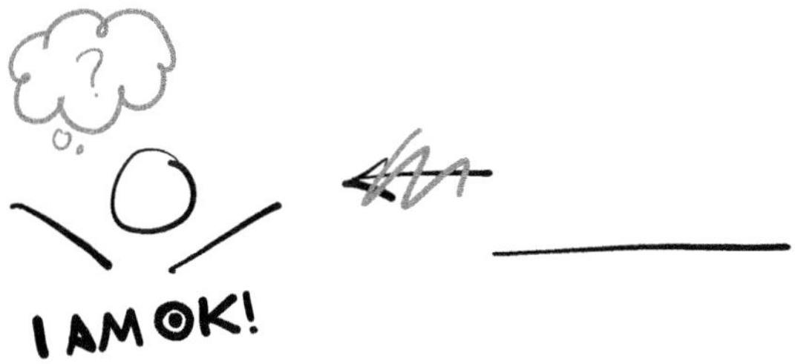

I find it helpful to think about the intelligent potential of our minds as being like electricity. Electricity has no preference as to whether you are using it to make a cup of tea or electrocute someone.

It rushes to power the direction we give it. In the same way, the neutral energy of our creative minds will solve the problems we give it, filling the time and space we allow it.

If the fundamental premise is illogical—*I will be ok if...*—the energy of our minds will flow to attend to the (wrong) 'problem'. It will never work. We are bound to struggle with life. I cannot stress this enough. We have input the wrong equation at the beginning of our calculation. It will not work, no matter what genius solutions we come up with. Whatever we create is based on an error. There will be no end of solutions to the wrong bloody problem.

When this happens a lot, we become confused and disheartened, realising we cannot control other people and the world—much as we try. Life makes no sense and feels terribly complicated. What are we supposed to do? We feel bad. What can help us?

We may not be able to thrive in this misunderstanding at all. Much like our ancestors must have felt, imagining someone or something could take away the sun, our capacity for life and to be ok seems terrifyingly unreliable.

This is why it's so unbelievably helpful to uncover a beautiful and perfect logic to the human experience. We have a new and stable foundation from which to create our lives. We CAN evolve.

We relax and begin to fall in love with life—instead of creating the living hell I did...

8.
CREATING HELL

What goes up must come down.
Isaac Newton

In my late teens, I became obsessed with making myself and my life look good to other people. I had completely lost sight of what actually felt good for me. This was my normal. I was at the mercy of the idea that I would be ok if I achieved my ideals. And if I didn't, *I was not ok*.

By my early twenties, I started to fall apart. Things that had previously made me feel better weren't working so well. I was doing them more and more.

I firmly believed that if there were less of me physically, that would be a good thing for everyone. Everything would be better if I slipped my little self through life more neatly and elegantly. No more mess. It had to all look good and be perfect. I had no idea I had made this up. This was simply my reality.

The now habitual management of my body became the problem itself. My disordered eating and relationship to my physical form made sense. I was trying to fix what I saw as broken. The punishing routine of starving and exercising was bad, but bulimia was the peak of the madness.

It had started in my late teens with something I only did every so often. It slowly morphed into a shameful double life. Something I did not want anyone else to know or see. I would have been mortified had anyone known.

This terrible secret added even more shame and disgust to the mental party. I was at war with my own body. My own private war I had waged, in my flat, alone—losing—night after night to throwing up. It was not even what I would call existing.

As I lay on the floor ashamed, alone and exhausted, I imagined I was going mad. Then I would get up. Go to work with a smile on my face. Until even pretending to be ok became impossible.

Paradoxically, it felt like I was doing something constructive even though it was ultimately so destructive. But frankly, it was a break from the constant thinking of how not-good-enough I was.

The eating felt like a release. It was nourishing and kind—permission to be indulgent. Then the purging was a correction, driven by my disgust at the indulgence. A breaking of those self-imposed rules. It had worked at first but then cascaded into a horrible, secret habit.

The weird solution I stumbled upon gave me some good feelings. I was in control, creating a momentary problem I could then fix. But it also gave me hell. It gave me everything and nothing. It was a total waste of a life. And I knew it.

Why do we do such strange things? How do we veer so far from the lives we want to live?

Finding ourselves doing crazy and illogical things is disturbing. It's like a loud, high-pitched, screeching alarm going off constantly in the background of our lives. I look back and feel lucky. My drug of choice, my war, was so insane that it was clear I needed help. I knew I was not ok, AND I did not know how to begin to be ok again.

The vicious cycle

Nowhere is it more evident that we are off track than in the nutty compulsions and habits we develop. The desire we have to use harmful substances and dangerous actions to numb ourselves or make us feel better temporarily. Be it a packet of biscuits, alcohol, pills or our screens. Sometimes we use repetitive behaviours to feel better—work, sex, cleaning, gambling, shopping or exercise. We do these things because they appear to make us feel good.

Most of us won't experience extreme addiction. Often what we struggle with settles down, without us ever understanding why we got so caught up, kinda lost it for a while and acted crazy.

Remember the relationship that drove you around the bend? You could not stop yourself behaving badly. You could not accept someone not wanting you. How about the job that kept you up, night after night? Those weeks you kept crying all the time. The knot in your stomach you felt for years. The way you had to wash your hands 50 times a day, or you could not rest until the house was spotless. Perhaps you went on a five-day alcohol or drug-fuelled binge of which you remember little. Or maybe you have experienced scary repetitive thinking about hurting yourself or others.

A times life can feel complex and overwhelming. We can gather evidence as to why we are uniquely rubbish, or other people are. We imagine all the reasons why we are not feeling or doing great. We will conjure up instances of all the times others have hurt us. All the things we have done wrong.

We become completely enmeshed in our personal experiences. There is nowhere to go and no relief because our paralysing and desperate beliefs about what we need to be ok remain unchallenged. We then live in the experience of these illogical and false beliefs about life—of course we don't feel all right!

We have an epic pity party and life does not look good at all. Then you add in all the crazy shit we do to try and feel better that isn't working, and you can see why life looks so horrible and pointless.

Addictions are entirely logical if we live from an illogical premise about life. It's what we do because nothing else seems to work any better. We are stuck.

Some of us desperately try to hold it all together so at least it doesn't look like it's all going wrong—even though it is. Others go into full-on malfunction mode. A human being not doing great, glitching away in the corner. Stuck in an inexplicable cycle of doing something insane over and over again.

We can't feel our innate wellbeing when we are caught up living in a horrifying and vicious cycle we have created of being, doing and having. And so it goes around, becoming more and more solid—more and more real. We have entangled ourselves in our dependencies to be ok. The entanglement is what we feel when we struggle.

Our thinking creates more feelings >>> more thinking >>> MORE FEELINGS.

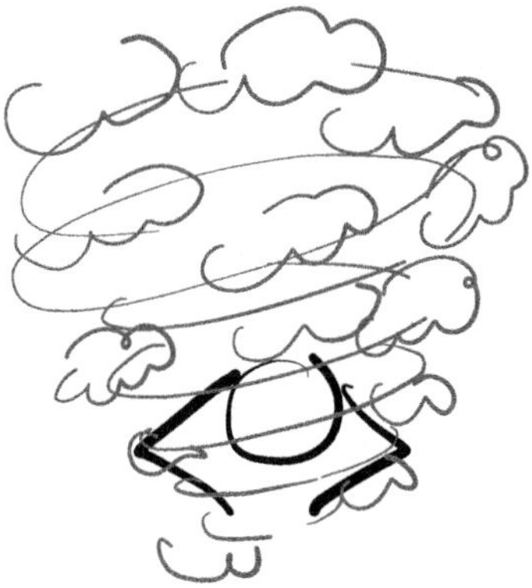

We go round and round in circles. We become disoriented. There seems no way out of our predicament. We need relief. We want to feel ok again. We will cut ourselves, make ourselves sick, starve ourselves or push our bodies to extremes with exercise and surgeons, who add things in or cut things out. We do push ourselves to achieve more or win the race and we will drive ourselves to get more knowledge, more money, more stuff or more fame.

Of course, the other viable option is simply zoning out. We get prescriptions for medication, drugs from our dealers and drink every single day. *Just to take the edge off. Just to feel ok again*. It does not really matter how we medicate ourselves, but **why**?

And what happens when it doesn't work anymore, or we need to do it more and more of the time? When the thing we do to feel better itself becomes another reason to feel bad?

We will try to transcend this human shite and get high as a kite. Naturally, spiritually or chemically. We want to fly high all the time.

Often these things do make us feel good or even super high. Problem is that it feels like flying until we hit the bloody floor again. Yes, what goes up must come down—Law of physics, I'm afraid.

There is a way it works for all of us. The amount of dependency and misunderstanding we have will exactly equal the consequential struggle. The highs will match the lows. We cannot know one without the other.

Medicating more often might seem like the only way out. I now understand our addictions and compulsions as so completely and utterly innocent. It's what we do when we don't know where our terrifying and out-of-control experience comes from. We want it to stop. Of course we do.

> You can't go back and change the beginning, but you can start where you are and change the ending.
>
> C. S. Lewis

To be in the throes of addiction is a demoralising and debilitating contradiction. It's madness. Hell.

If you are struggling in this way, no words can express the compassion I have for you. Where you are, I have been. The struggle is real. I have written this book for you because there is hope my friend.

No matter how worn out and used up you have been feeling. There is only one place you are ok, exactly as you are. Here, in this very moment, you CAN thrive and be well. In this place, you can recover and overcome anything.

Let's reorientate you. You have veered off track from the path where you are blessed with everything you need. Why? Because you innocently believe a version of *I will be ok if...*

This mistaken idea means you will struggle. The good news is that you can return to being ok at any time, no matter how off track and stuck you feel.

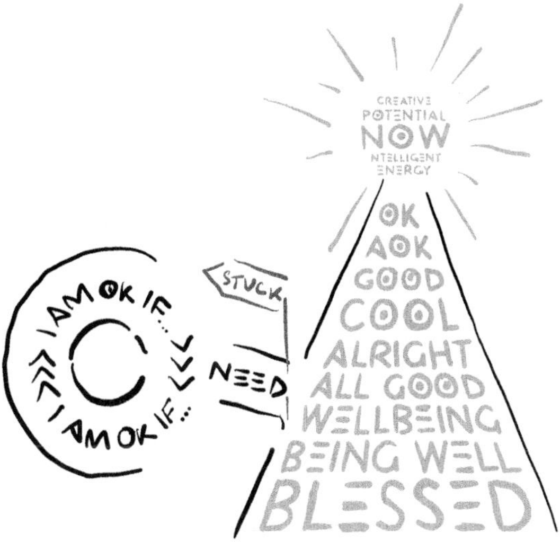

The peace we all crave is only ever found in *being*. Right now, as you read this line. This is where we have been blessed with everything we need. This is the only place you can finally put down the heavy burden you have carried. You don't need to do that anymore.

We all can become less dependent when we orient ourselves around our innate mental health. We don't need to white-knuckle our compulsive behaviours. We don't need all the answers right now. When we get present, a natural openness to new ways of being is available.

Healing does not come from hating yourself. Healing comes from love. And what is love? Looks to me like love is simply the generation of powerful and positive connections—within yourself, with other people and with the world. That's it.

You CAN create one simple positive connection. Make one simple healthy choice and take one small next step. There is only ever the potential to act in this exact moment. Here we are all only ever up against the same thing.

When we are present, life becomes less personal and way more abundant than it may have seemed.

9.

IT'S NOT PERSONAL

I am not crazy, my reality is just different from yours.

Cheshire Cat, Alice's Adventures in Wonderland

I know; life feels pretty personal. Especially when it's extreme, either going really well (*aren't we clever and brilliant)* OR really badly *(it's all my fault / it's all your fault!).* But the illusion of life is real and so it should be.

It's a bit like watching a movie. We can get so engrossed in the film, gasp with delight, cringe with embarrassment, physically move from danger, cry sad tears. Well, I do anyway. I allow myself to go on a ride and enjoy the special effects. Even a scary, horrifying or tragic ride. Why? Because I know it's a movie. Life is similar. When we know we create our experience, there is so much potential to marvel at it AND enjoy it much more than we do.

Life will inevitably suck at times but taking it personally is optional. What a revelation. This has done wonders for me—and those around me.

Without really knowing it, most of us are skipping down the yellow brick road of life much of the time. We are just doing the do, living and being, not worrying or stressing about it. Taking each step, blessed with inspiration and creativity.

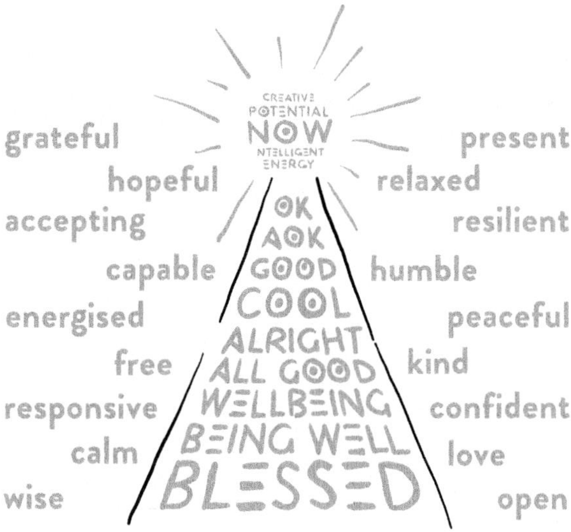

Deciding *I'm going home now. I'll take this route today. Oooo, what shall I eat tonight? Hmmmm. Pasta! *Chooses favourite pasta, add water, boil the pot, drain it* Time for a shower. Do me teeth. Get to bed. Set the alarm... Zzzz.*

Subconsciously we make choice after mundane choice. These dictate our actions, which create the next hour, day, week, year or decade—a lifetime. We don't consider how these simple choices and actions keep us alive. We overlook entirely the genius within us that allows us to do complex tasks with ease. It's more compelling to focus on where we feel off and not appreciate the many areas of our lives where we are ok. For me too.

When we veer off track, boy do we feel it. Stressed is when being blessed has become dependent on something external. We take a detour off our blessed path into a path of resistance when something looks real to us that isn't.

I feel bad—*I need to do more / I want to have more / I must change something* to be ok. There is a *Blessed if... Blessed when... Blessed because...* We look for blessings outside of us, forgetting that being blessed is **who we are.**

We have simply veered off track, down little paths where we meet all our beliefs about our life and what we need to be ok. Repetitive areas we struggle with can awaken us to where we are at.

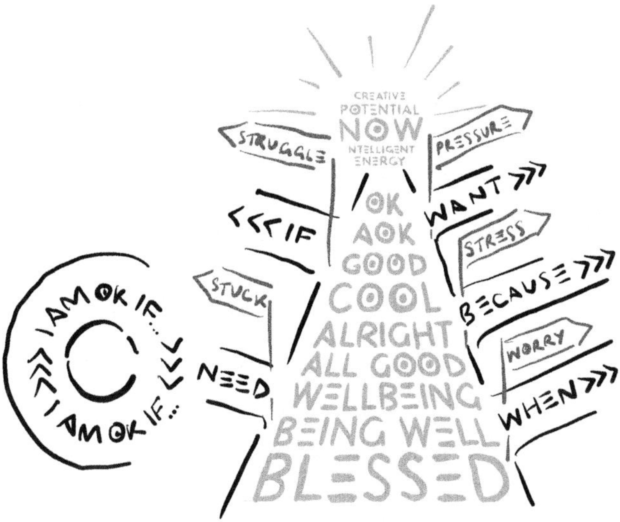

We feel it when we are off. We don't feel ok. Feelings of worry, stress and pressure are literal signposts to help us navigate life and show us where we have veered off track. Feelings aren't a source of factual information about the world. Feelings are generated within us and reflect what we think.

A good analogy for this can be found in a car. All cars fundamentally work the same way. So when a light comes on the car's dashboard, be it green, amber or flashing red, would you open the window and look outside for the source of the problem? Would you shout at a passer-by, *Oi mate! What have you done to my car? You made my light come on!*

No. That would be an irrational thing to do. The warning light tells you what is going on *inside* your car; in the same way, a feeling illuminates what is on your mind. Our feelings helpfully alert us to what we are thinking; they point us back to our inner reality. Now we have a choice.

What looks true for us about life right now? What is available when we step out of our ideas about what we need?

The neutrality this curiosity requires brings us right back on track, where we don't *need* to know. Where nothing *needs* to change and we don't *need* to do better.

Remember, the sun is always there even if we cannot see it. We can begin to understand what is happening within us and how to come home. When we start to appreciate this truth in our own lives, we see it is true for other people too.

Other people

Let's face it, what gets our backs up and challenges us the most is other people. Our partners, families, kids, parents, teammates, teachers, bosses, work colleagues, friends and those difficult people in our lives.

What can we do about them? Especially the ones who drive us nuts.

It really feels like we feel so bad because of someone else. *Nah, nothing to do with me; it's all someone else's fault. It's my parent's fault. My family should have... My partner needs to... My friends should... My boss must...*

We fill up with feelings of victimisation, anger, regret and even vengeance. We feel powerless; *They must change for us to be ok again—right?*

But of course, rarely do people do what we think they should. I know it's so annoying. It can feel so unbearable and unjust to us. But guess what? People are unreliable because they struggle with life the same way we do. We all do stupid things and make bad decisions when we don't think we are ok. The only thing we can do is ascertain where we are at. Are we living from a mistaken idea about life? *I am only alright if...*

Or do we know we are ok no matter what? Are we on the blessed or stressed path?

Recently my four-year-old daughter, Didi, came to me and tapped me on the arm. "Mummy!" She whispered. "Yessssss", I murmured, not looking up. "A boy is being mean to me at school." That got my attention. I turned to her and looked at her lovely little face. I hugged her. *Awww.*

Luckily, I had just been writing about the innocence of bad behaviour. I was curious. "Is he being mean to you? Or is he being mean to everyone?" I asked.

"Everyone! Even the teachers know he is mean!" she explained, wide-eyed.

I asked her, "Do you think he is being mean because he feels good inside or bad?" Without missing a beat, she replied, "bad". We held each other's gaze and simply nodded. She understood.

Page for Reflection

We just don't tend to do very well when we feel bad. We go into the world looking to get better feelings by hook or by crook.

Don't get me wrong; I explained all the practical things she could do if he continued to be mean. There is no need to endure the effects of other people's bad behaviour.

But as we realise our own misunderstandings in life, we will take it less personally when other people behave badly. We are less attached to outcomes. They don't need to change for us to know we are ok. This takes a lot off our minds and creates space for how best to respond and look after ourselves.

Sometimes though, it's hard to see this when we feel bad, the lights are out and the world feels dark and scary. So in an ideal world, we would look for the answers to life when the lights are on. When we are not in the darkness of a whole heap of pain and overthinking. So, from a more spacious and settled down place, let's consider what **we believe** about our relationships?

> If someone comes along and shoots an arrow into your heart, it's fruitless to stand there and yell at the person. It would be much better to turn your attention to the fact that there's an arrow in your heart.
>
> Pema Chödrön

Do we believe it is other people that make us feel good? That they must behave a certain way for us to be ok? Most of us imagine relationships are a transaction—you need to make me feel good and I need to make you feel good.

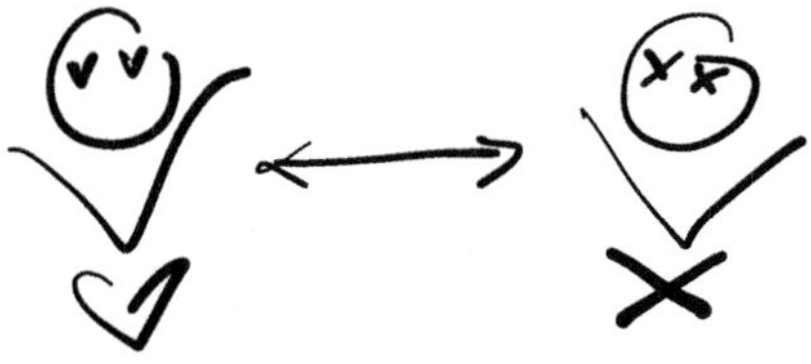

For example, I believe my partner makes me feel secure, loved, loving and excited. I now *need* my partner so I can feel these feelings. I have developed a dependency which means I will struggle in my relationship. Remember, *what goes up must come down.*

When my partner inevitably does not make me feel good, I will feel insecure. I need my partner to make me feel ok again. Which they may or may not be willing to do. I am reliant on them; I *need* them to change or give me something to feel better again. *Aaaargh.*

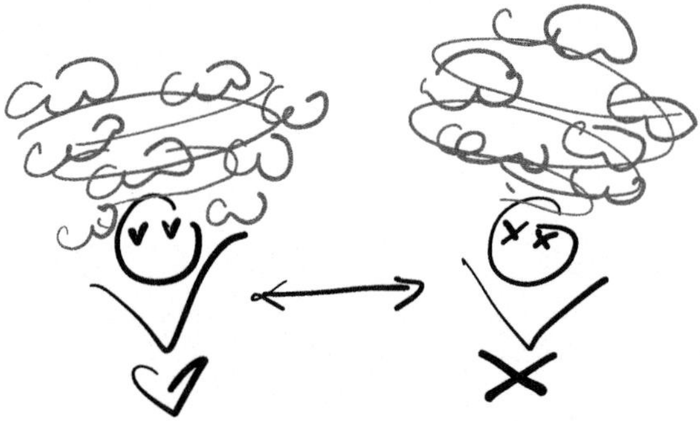

We will feel the insecurity created by these misunderstandings infiltrate our lives. Not just in our closest relationships but in every relationship we have. The amount we struggle is directly correlated to the extent we believe other people need to do what we think they should do for us to be ok. Do we realise our independent capacity to be well?

If we give others the power to *make us* feel good, they inevitably have the power to make us feel bad. This causes so much human struggle and unnecessary suffering.

We give our power away to people who probably don't even want that power over us. Who feel as confused as we do about life and what we are asking of them, however much they love us. Because I cannot emphasise this enough: people are unreliable. I am unreliable.

Yup. I don't mean to be. My kids don't know if I will ignore the filthy kitchen or shout at them for it. There are many variables as to why I may or may not shout today. Am I feeling tired, hungry, fed up or off-track myself? It's entirely possible I may be all these things at once, which massively increases the probability of me losing it. So no, we don't want to rely on others for our ok-ness because they may or may not feel ok themselves.

There will surely be times for us all when we feel troubled by other people. How easily can a simple situation have us in its grip and wake us at night? It always amazes me how quickly a deep insecurity can set upon us from which none of us is immune.

Maybe we disagree with someone, after which we replay conversations and arguments in our heads for days. We anxiously try to work out what happened and how we can feel right again. Ah yes, nothing like needing to be 'right' and therefore others to be 'wrong' to cause unnecessary suffering for all involved. Life instantly becomes exceedingly personal and limited for us. Naturally we become defensive. We no longer feel secure and ok.

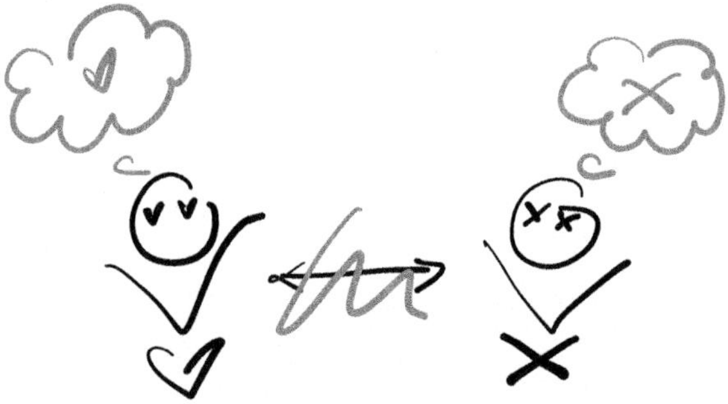

When this happens what can we do about it? Again, it's so good to know our feelings will helpfully illuminate where we are at. What is going on for us? What exactly is the thinking creating these perturbing feelings? When we get curious and begin to settle down, we can gain clarity. Now there is the potential to realise that the metaphorical arrows we believe are attaching us do not exist.

These 'arrows' can look so beautiful, especially in our closest relationships—*You make me feel so loved and special. You are my everything. I am nothing without you...* But the imagined arrows straight into our 'hearts' creating our loving feelings are actually the reason we hurt in relationships and become insecure. If we are struggling with someone else, what do we believe we *need* to be ok right now? Have we outsourced our ok-ness to them? If so, we are going to fill up with ideas of how to manipulate and control them to create feelings within them. This wont go well and is the misunderstanding that leads to all conflict.

When we, as individuals, become more curious about our own struggles—this will help untangle us all—one human at a time. Take a moment. Reflect, *hold on, where am I at? What's going on for me? Do I know I am ok?*

Page for Reflection

We make the rules.

I realise it may feel like there are some urgent situations in the world we *must* address. But perhaps our biggest problem is that no one can agree what the problems are, let alone the solutions. As usual, we just can't reach a consensus on who needs to do what for us all to be ok.

Yes, humans have done things in the past that do not work, they may have worked once or never have worked, but they were the best we had with the beliefs and ideas we held. Like our ancestors' sacrifices to the Gods to save the sun, change happens. Thankfully we are evolving, both personally and collectively.

Yet we seem bound to keep facing the same old problem—each other: *those people over there and their bad ideas. Let's cancel them. Fight them. Destroy them!* So important to pay attention to OUR angry feelings.

We believe we are right, SO they must be wrong (x=y). The ideas behind our righteous feelings are based on our own innocent misunderstanding of life. We create our lives based on our deepest but invisible beliefs about who we are, how others must behave and how the world should be.

Most of us have an idea that ALL humans need to behave a certain way and do certain things to be good and have a good life. *Obviously! Duh—then we will ALL be ok.*

We are taught some version of this by our parents, caregivers, friends, schools and work environments. This is how life works. If you do it 'right', you will be all good.

We literally create rules; then, we need other people to play by our rules. People should agree with us or be polite / kind / tidy / welcoming / honest etc. When people don't behave that way, they have challenged our fundamental ideas about what should or needs to happen. We inescapably get angry and frustrated. We throw our hands in the air incredulously. *What's the matter with them? Unbelievable!*

> The highest activity a human being can attain is learning for understanding, because to understand is to be free.
>
> Baruch Spinoza

When we do not understand what is creating our experience, we definitely can't see it for others. When people around us get out of sorts, angry or upset, we often mirror them, which is not just illogical but unbelievably unhelpful. Suddenly we find ourselves screaming at someone to calm down. *Well, I'm angry because you're angry!*

I was raised with the idea that *if you don't have anything nice to say, don't say it.* My husband was not raised with this idea. I believed he was wrong when he said whatever was true for him. I felt angry at his truth. *Hmmmm.*

You see, I *need* people to be 'nice' for me to be ok, whereas he does not. It was confusing. I was offended and triggered when he didn't conform to my ideas about being 'nice'. *Whoa—That' not nice! You need to change!*

And of course, for us all, when we think you are the problem—we need to do something about you. *You have to feel sorry! You must change!* We imagine other people have the power to take away our ok-ness and capacity to thrive. They *make* us feel bad.

We will reliably be on the road of resistance and conflict. Marching firmly down the stressed road where we need other people to change, NOW preferably.

We develop specific ideas about the world and we need others to see life as we do—so we can all be ok. *The road to hell is indeed paved with good intentions.*

The experience we create is so predictable. If we believe we are not ok, or our people or loved ones are not ok, our intelligent psychological system will generate ideas about what needs to happen. These ideas can be both super-creative AND unbearably damaging. After all, this is the same creative genius that produces all hate too. This is perhaps the simplest explanation for all 'evil'. Our minds will fill up with solutions to the problem of you. *Something MUST be done about YOU!*

We are right and we don't like your way of being. *It's all YOUR fault I feel bad. I am not ok!?* We feel threatened by your opinion. *How dare you say that!?* We feel judgemental and critical. *Are you stupid!? How dare you think that?* We shut down and can't bear to listen to you. We simply don't respect your ideas so communication is off the table.

We will talk badly about you to your face or behind your back. We cannot stop ourselves. These triggering and angry feelings reflect our illogical thinking.

In this state, we cannot appreciate diversity and difference. We are stuck. And the more we believe that you doing something differently can make us ok again, the more we are bound to live a life of blame and fear.

We feel insecure and will constantly catastrophise potential outcomes. *It's a disaster! I am never going to be ok again! We are all doomed.* This is amplified when we discover like-minded people and form groups. When everyone is fighting to protect their version of reality, life becomes a literal disaster zone. We fight and defend what we believe in, but do we really interrogate these beliefs?

If we are angry with others, can WE see there are other perspectives available? If not, then maybe the problem is not what we think it is?

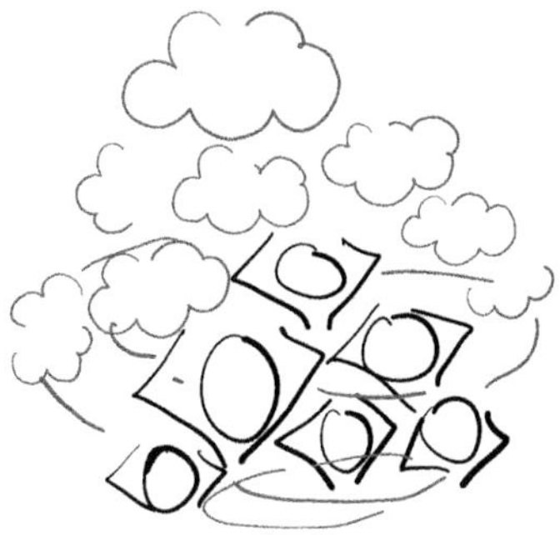

WE ARE OK IF…

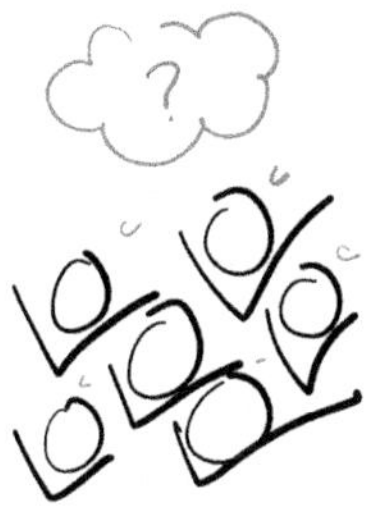

WE ARE OK.

We are following an ill-making logic that our wellbeing is reliant on someone else. Can you see how we are bound to react from this place? Unnecessary human tragedy, suffering and misery WILL occur until we can find neutrality within ourselves. This is essential for us to understand so we stop pointing fingers at others.

We don't struggle because people have different ideas or beliefs; we struggle because of the beliefs we have created. *What reality are WE creating? What do we want? What do we think we need to be ok?*

These simple enquiries can help release us from the dependencies and entanglements that continuously separate us. We are the same. We will all strive to be right, be better, have more and do more when we don't know that we already have what we are looking for.

When we truly appreciate our own innocent misunderstandings, we can see them in other people. We know they too, are blessed with innate health, resilience and wisdom. When we come from that knowing, full of compassion and love, we are equals. We don't need to make others wrong so we can be right. We don't need to change other people for us to be ok.

The possibility to enjoy and value the diversity of our minds is available. Are we in such a rush that we cannot take the time to stop and listen for the wisdom and reasoning of another? If we have trouble connecting to others we can get curious, *what do I think I need to be ok? What do they think they need to be ok?* There is always an opportunity to listen to understand, because it is OUR presence that will bring peace.

We have found a beautiful neutrality in our experience. It IS possible. **Peace in the world is an inside job.**

10.

BEING OK IS AN INSIDE JOB

When I let go of what I am,
I become what I might be.

Lao Tzu

So how can we help others? How do we help the world? When we learn how we work, it makes sense to turn within, knowing that the peace we yearn for is only found inside us. It's not personal but universal.

However, it can be hard to recognise and appreciate the struggle of others. In the same way, people often don't sympathise with us because our struggles may look silly or illogical to them.

When we finally share the source of our woes, others can sensibly advise us... *Come on; it will be ok!* They may help us come up with ideas and solutions to our problems. Or suggest we focus on something else. *You must look at all the things going well in your life.* We may even get a stern and unsympathetic shake of the head; *get a grip!*

Or my least fave—*We are not sent anything we can't handle.* The sentiment of a person who just ain't struggling like we are right now. *Ummmmm—hello!? I can't bloody handle it??? That's why I am talking to you!?*

What helps us is someone who can listen and hold our ok-ness when we can't see it. Who will trust us to find our wisdom without taking over and telling us what to do. Who will help us uncover our own, reliable source of wellbeing that will sustain us throughout our lives.

I was working with a beautiful, vibrant and creative young woman recently. She told me that she always had to get the last word. We laughed.

"I have to be right and you have to know it!" She grinned at me shyly. This was in the middle of a conversation about how someone at work had upset her. She had been practising what she would say in response for days—changing her mind, settling on something and then changing her mind again. She had been talking to herself all week. (FYI, A pretty good red flag that we are off track)

I asked her, "What do you want from this girl?"

She raised an eyebrow. "She needs to know Kat! I am right." Her mischievous eyes were twinkling contagiously.

"I hear you", I said. "But why does her knowing you are right matter?"

Unsure, she wrinkled her nose. I went on, "Look, she does not sound like she is being very nice, but that's her problem. I am more interested in you spending the whole week having conversations and arguments in your head? That's your problem. What do you feel like you need?"

We gazed at each other in open curiosity.

"I need her to know I am right and I need her to acknowledge that I am not wrong" she carefully worked it through. I nodded encouragingly.

She slowed down a bit. "I need to show them they are not right and that I am not wrong. I need them to know that. I need to know it's not my fault". She was quiet. "When my dad left when I was younger, I needed to know it was not my fault. That there's not something wrong with me."

I nodded in response, tears brimming. It was a powerful moment. Her wisdom and curiosity had brought her home.

What do we think we need? What is it we feel we are lacking? What belief have we developed that we are unconsciously basing our lives on?

Can you see the absolute innocence behind the beliefs and burdens we carry with us through life? Going around in circles, trying to get our needs met. We don't see any choice, doing the same things hoping for different results, falling back into our vicious cycle.

We don't need to feel bad all the time; we can gently allow ourselves to get curious. *Why am I feeling so insecure / jealous / out of sorts / stressed? Why am I talking to this person in my imagination? WHAT DO I WANT?*

If you are struggling with a specific circumstance or issue, it may be beneficial to talk it through with someone who can help you hear your wisdom and health. Usually, we just want to be seen, heard or valued, especially if we feel rejected. We want to be loved. Our deepest fear is that in our mess, we are unlovable. That what we do and have done makes us not ok. Messy. Wrong. Useless. Rejection is more evidence that there must be something wrong with us.

We don't feel ok and become entangled with our personal experience—what's going on for us—and live in that obsession. We can't pull out to a neutral place beyond the personal, where a different perspective is available.

We light up when we finally understand there is nothing wrong with us. When we finally realise we are not uniquely flawed. That we just innocently misunderstood how life worked. We can appreciate that there is a way in which all humans work, which helps us make sense of our own experience.

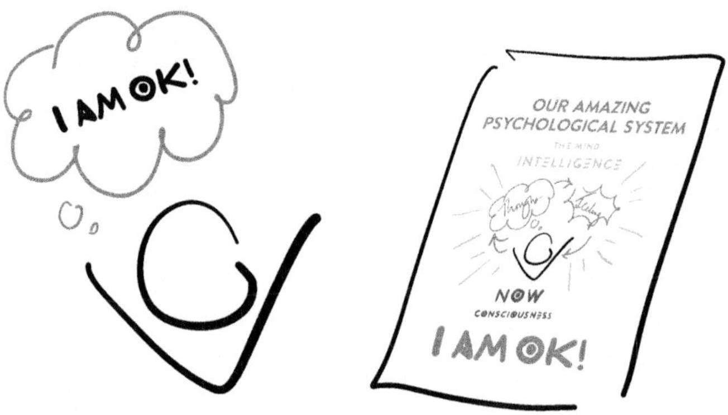

When we know we are ok; we feel secure; this allows for ease and simplicity in our experience. No matter how others are being, we are free and able to listen. We are open and interested in diverse ideas and the wisdom of others. We don't need to see things the same way. There is no need to jump in and convince you that *I am right and you are wrong.* This allows us to communicate with each other.

No one will agree with us on everything, which is cool because that is how we evolve. We can be honest yet respectful of others' opinions, and who knows? We may even learn something new! We can stop wasting our valuable time on earth pointing our fingers. We know we can only ever find love, hope and security within ourselves. It is 100% an inside job. AND we don't need to do anything, just relax back into being.

Creating the change in our lives and the world we would like is on us, my lovely new friend. We don't want to wait for someone to do it for us because, unless we are a small child or live in a fairytale, no one is coming to save us. I know, it sucks. But this is not the bitter pill it may appear to be. We don't need anyone to save us. Some people may show up and help us out a lot, which is great, but DO NOT rely on it or wait for it. Remember how we are all up against the same thing?

There will be times we get confused and imagine that how well we do is personal. We believe **who we are** is determined by all the external factors outside us and how we react to them. We are being taught that our capacity to be ok is dependent on where we are born, our families, our circumstances, how we look, our personalities and what relationships or influence we have. It seems complex and precarious.

Thank goodness it's not. It's very simple.

Who I am

When we are born, there is a little tag tied on our wrist or foot with our family name on. This is so we don't get confused with another little new being. Using language to describe ourselves or others can be helpful, but do words tell us who we are?

I am often struck by how much we want to define ourselves; this *is who I am*—creating an identity checklist. But I love to ask people I am working with, who are struggling with some aspect of their identity, "Do you need to decide this right now, at this exact moment? Or even today?"

Let's do a little exercise. How have you labelled yourself or been labelled by others?

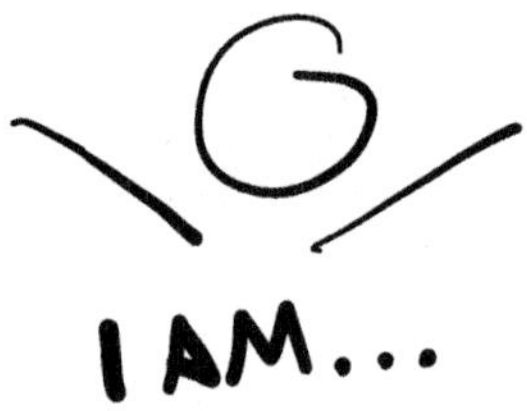

Please take a moment to reflect: write, *I am...* in the middle of a page, ideally, under a little sketch of yourself. Then around it, write out some of the labels you have been given in your life. You may have been given them by others or created them yourself.

Start with your name and some positive labels you attribute to yourself or that other people have given you.

I am... *a good listener / kind / thoughtful / creative / loving / brave / smart / cool.*

Try to think of some less 'positive' ones too.

I am... *shy / crazy / boring / unlucky / a nightmare / selfish / a control freak / nerdy / an idiot / perfectionist / demanding / untidy.* Here is my example.

I am... *relaxed / demanding / creative / shy / happy / honest / opinionated.*

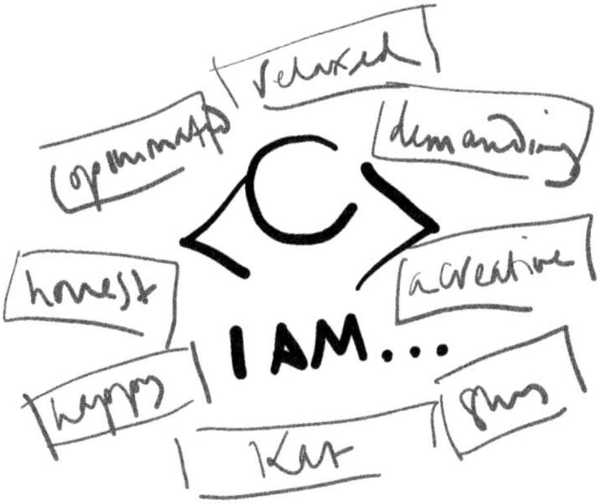

What are yours?
I am...

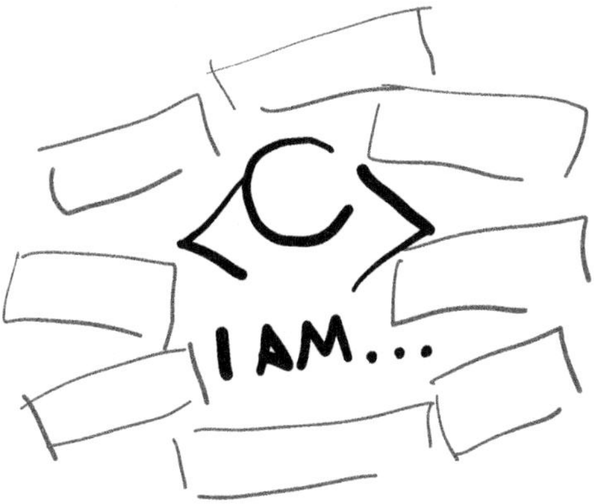

Once you have done this, choose a 'positive' and a 'negative' label that feels juicy. For example, 'honest' and 'shy'.

Page for Reflection

Ask yourself these questions for each label you choose to explore:

- **Do you like being this label?** (Eg. Do you like being shy?)
- **Do you always feel this way? All day every day?**
- **Was there ever a time when you did not feel this?**
- **Were you born with this label?**
- **Can I take this label from you and put it on the table right now? Why not?**
- **Who would you be without this label?**
- **And finally, would you be willing to let this label go?**

I love this exercise. By questioning the assumptions we make about ourselves and others, we can start to see how real our labels are. Of course, we can't put our labels on the table. They are not solid; they don't exist. They are ideas.

We can cling to them and wear them like a badge of honour, *I know, I am so clever* or a cloak of protection, *Well I'm just shy so I can't...* Or perhaps a get out of jail free card; I *just had to tell you—you look terrible because I am soooo honest.*

Many of us will spend our lives using limiting beliefs about ourselves as an excuse to stay small. Especially when we have developed ideas like *I am an idiot. I can't do anything right. I am a failure. There is something wrong with me.* They seem true and real, and we see life through this limiting lens.

Labelling ourselves and other people is something we do to simplify things, but labels don't tell us who we are. They are a way we are being—sometimes. Perhaps they have become habitual, or we've become invested in them, but when we question our labels, we can take them less seriously. We can wear them more lightly, knowing they are a temporary creation of our minds.

Who would we be without our labels? Who are we?

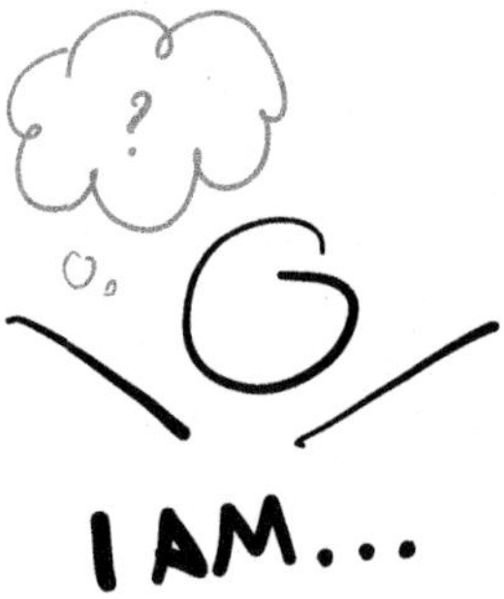

We are free. You are free. I am free—to just be me! As I am right now, as we are in this moment, however that shows up. We can be open to evolving and changing our minds. We don't need to bring a whole load of solid ideas and fixed expectations to life. We don't need to limit ourselves and other people by ticking boxes. This is not who we are.

All our potential becomes available as we release the layers of ideas and beliefs that cloud our true and expansive nature. We can let life unfold from a deep understanding that we are innately well. A unique expression of one divine and unifying thing. This is who we are.

No matter where we were born or what we have done, we each have the same warm glowing sun within, a neutral yet infinite part of us no one can take away.

We have finally found the security we crave was within us all along, which makes sense because we never could find it out there in life.

11.
PLAYING IN THE UNKNOWN

We suffer more often in imagination than in reality.

Lucius Annaeus Seneca

There is no escaping that life can be brutal and many of us will suffer the effects of it. Perhaps there is extreme danger; we are unwell or do not have enough food or shelter. There may well be natural disasters, ill health, accidents, abuse, attack, war and of course, we will all face eventual death.

For all of us, there will be tragedies and challenges in life. However, we can only experience these things as they happen now, where we can attend to our necessary and pressing needs. This may go well or not. We will suffer the effects of physical lack or danger. But this is not struggling; this is surviving. We will generate ideas about what to do and how to help ourselves or others.

We have evolved to respond to our immediate circumstances. If some crazy flying bat flew into your room right now, you would defend yourself instinctively because we have the most genius survival reflexes. We aren't even conscious of them until after the fact. We often call this our fight or flight response.

Instantly, a natural process in our bodies floods us with the chemicals we need to trigger alertness and action. Adrenaline pumps us up to react to dangerous and threatening situations. This surge of energy is designed to help us and give us the best chance of survival possible.

One snowy day I was in the car with my son. I turned onto a road that developed into a steep hill. At the end of this hill, you had to turn left or right or drive straight into the house at the end of the road. Quite by surprise, halfway down this hill, I completely lost all control of my car when we hit ice. I became calm as we skated serenely down towards the junction. To this day, I could not tell you exactly what I did. Something like slam the accelerator, pull the handbrake and turn the steering wheel as far as it would go. I know what I did made no sense to me afterwards, but my instinctive reaction worked. The wheels picked up friction and prevented us from gatecrashing someone's front room. That is responsiveness.

'I didn't have time to think', we often say in these situations. What we mean is that we didn't have time to think twice or overthink it. We do what makes *sense* to us. So, if we make it out alive, it's because the innate intelligent systems within have given us the best shot at surviving.

The struggle is not real (but it sure is helpful!)

Struggle will only be found in the assessment, analysis and perceived implications of our situation. What meaning we create and attach to it. When we don't accept what has happened or why, we may begin to feel insecure and unsafe.

If we judge how it happened, we may feel useless, broken, unequipped, victimised or hopeless.

Stories have been told throughout time of ordinary people who kept going in the face of terrible circumstances and physical suffering. We understand this is an impressive feat that perhaps—just maybe—we are all equally capable of. And we are, our brain is designed to take care of us and keep us safe.

Unfortunately, this survival mechanism and full-body response can kick in when we are not actually in danger, as we sit in a traffic jam, answer a sh*tty email or get stuck on a call with an automated service provider. *Grrrr.* All the energy in our body responds to a whole lot of outraged thinking. Anger is a sign that we believe we are being threatened.

Our bodies flood with stress hormones that create an instant response. Our heart rate quickens, muscles tense and we may even start to sweat. We are ready. Something needs to happen right now. We are about to dive into action. *Uh oh.* Remember our dashboard?

It is hard to step back when the adrenaline has already kicked in but getting angry doesn't work and most often just makes us feel worse about ourselves and any damage we may have caused.

Some things look threatening to us that aren't. Some things look like they can take away our wellbeing that cannot. We are going to overreact when we perceive a threat to our being. Note the word *perceive.* When we think we are not ok, we have no choice but to react. This is good to know. Anger is not a sign that the 'idiot' on the phone is, in fact, an idiot; it is a sign we are off track. Maybe make that call or send our reply to the email later, when we are not so pumped up?

Do you feel angry sometimes? It would be interesting to consider a situation where you regularly get mad. Where and when do you get angry? Put it on the line. This will help you back to clarity. What exactly are you thinking? What about it makes you mad? Write it out and explore the ideas that create your angry feelings. Why are you angry? What do you feel you need to be ok?

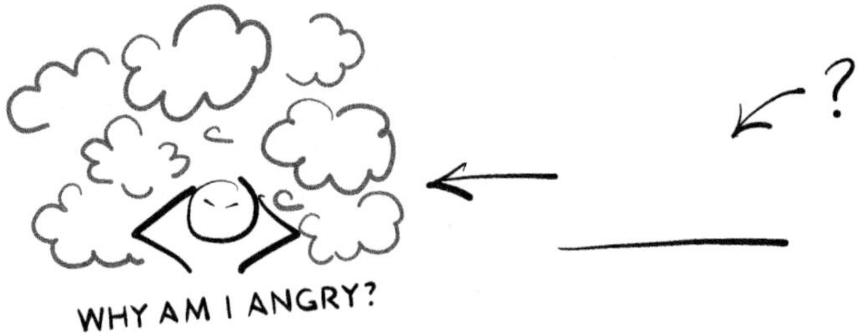

The majority of us aren't taught about our extraordinary minds. It's easy to grow up without understanding that we are creating our lives and entire reality ALL the time. Mostly we are directed away from our natural creativity, taught to respond to life in a way that will inevitably involve unnecessary struggle.

We find ourselves standing at a doorway, frantically pulling and pushing at it. Panicking, we can't get out. *This damn door! Get me outta here! It's stuck!? Is this me? Am I going mad?*

Oh, we suddenly realise sheepishly, this is a sliding door. *That's how it works.* So too, can we easily open a metaphorical door to new ways of being.

The illusion of life is real and we can get confused, but we reach out for help because we know we are struggling unnecessarily. We feel stuck and caught up like someone has tied us up in knots. We can't seem to free ourselves but

Page for Reflection

suspect it surely does not need to be this way. We are open to learning something we don't already know.

We are only ever as stuck as we think. Our struggle is a blessing in disguise, helpfully showing us where we have veered off the yellow brick road and directing us back home to the warming rays of our inner sun. All that was needed was a little nudge back on track—a little curiosity.

We can develop a deep trust that we have found security within. We are full of potential to navigate our lives. The starting point is knowing where we are at—is NOT who we are. This is so hopeful. There will be some beliefs about what you need and not getting that will be helpful to see.

Hope is found in this dance between what we know and don't know. Our struggle looks real because it is our reality—at this moment. As we become more confident in our innate human capabilities, we are no longer looking to feel better when we feel bad but to understand why we felt bad in the first place. Struggle becomes more optional. We know we are too blessed to be stressed. Blessed not by what we do and have, but in our very being.

Life is not against us; life is happening FOR us.

> The whole world is a series of miracles, but we're so used to them we call them ordinary things.
>
> Hans Christian Andersen

The first time I understood life to be a bit less certain than I had imagined but way more magical was as a young teenager. I was sitting in my dad's huge old, grey tank of a car. The radio was playing an interview with an Irish comedian. I have no idea who he was, but he opened my eyes to a bigger picture of life. Here follows what I heard, which has stayed with me for 25 years.

"I hear you don't send your kids to school?" asked the interviewer. (Hard to imagine what made my teenage ears prick up at this part of the conversation.)

"Nooo. I do not want to send my kids to school," replied his melodic Irish lilt.

"Why ever not?" replied the incredulous interviewer in his clipped BBC voice.

"They want to teach my kids rationality. And I don't want my kids learning rationality," he said triumphantly.

The host and I chuckled; you had to. I instantly liked this guy after 10 seconds.

"Whatever is wrong with rationality?" the host mused, humouring his guest.

And here, stating the obvious – each word passionate, emphatic and in one long breath – is the epic reply:

"WE. ARE. ON. A. BALL. FLOATING. IN. THE. BLACK. ABYSS.—WE. DON'T. KNOW. WHAT. WE'RE. DOING. OR. WHY. WE'RE. HERE."

Silence. "And that's why I don't want my kids learning rationality," he concluded.

I didn't hear any more of the conversation. I was way too busy with the heavens opening. The bright light of pure truth descended into my dimly lit world. **Ahhhhhhhhhh*

I looked at my dad, incredulous. "Did you hear that?"

"Yes," he replied, not averting his eyes from the road. It was clear the heavens had not opened for him in quite the same way.

I sat quietly, digesting what I had heard. My first red pill. It remains one of the only times I have ever heard anyone talk about the biggest and simplest picture of our earthly predicament. A world view that finally sparked my imagination and made perfect sense.

I have since embellished this idea further and come to see it as even more comical. More ludicrous. Technically, we are all kicking back somewhere on a piece of broken crust, that somehow still encapsulates a molten ball of fire. Which itself appears to be precariously teetering in time, between either rolling off into the black abyss or being drawn towards another giant exploding ball of fire.

We are still none the wiser as to what the hell we are doing here or why. We tend not to think about it.

Perhaps for some, the big picture may feel scary? For me, it instantly calms the personal experience of my mind and like any grand vista, offers precious perspective. Who doesn't gaze up at the stars and feel the expansive nature of life? We humans have way more in common than difference, just doing the best we can on this crazy old ball.

Creativity begins in wonder

When we zoom out, we can see that our greatest fears and insecurities are unnecessary. Life is precarious; change and uncertainty are constant. Nothing stays the same. We are in a state of continuous evolution, physically and mentally.

It is our relationship with not knowing that defines our experience. We can either embrace the mystery of what will happen next or resist it. We have free will. How our lives go is our responsibility—literally response-ability. Our innate ability to respond.

A mind that is not filled up with the endless possibilities of change, and all the futile *shoulda / woulda / coulda's,* is a responsive mind. A mind in turmoil, mulling over all the ways it *should* be doing better or *needs* to change, is an entangled busy mind. A mind thinking about solving a problem—not a mind solving a problem. Thinking about creating but not creating.

Our new thinking on the problems of being human occurs from a free and quiet mind. If we become stuck, we can ascertain what is happening for us. *Hold on... what is the actual problem I am trying to solve here? What do I want or need?*

I recently tidied my room and working at my desk was an option again. The room was no longer chaotic; there was space to be in it. This is a good analogy for our minds. There is no space to be present when we have a cluttered and busy mind full of misguided beliefs and patterns.

We can spend time enjoying the intellectual capacity of our minds and the minds of others. But our new ideas mostly occur to us out of the blue.

Soaking ourselves in knowledge, striving for truth, researching our history and understanding how things work is essential. But we rarely get new ideas by thinking harder.

'Eureka!' Cried the mathematician Archimedes as he jumped up naked, having solved the problem of how to measure volume whilst enjoying a soak in the tub.

How often have you been struggling with something, even something silly, and an idea popped into your head? *Ping*. Maybe when you were in the shower, walking, cooking, driving... Perhaps when you were explaining the problem to someone else.

This is not random. New ideas and fresh thinking do not come from what we already know. New ideas came from an unedited, curious and quieter mind. There is space to explore. We open a metaphorical door to possibility.

Is this true? Is this possible? Ooooo, I wonder if...? Imagine if...? This line of enquiry creates a gap for the infinite and intelligent potential energy of life to flow through us. It is not on us. Our minds will naturally conceive solutions. We can then take practical steps to birth the creations of our minds into physical form—one simple step at a time.

Creativity begins with wonder and a good sprinkle of humility on top. How does earth orientate around a burning ball of fire and become full of life? How does the seed know to grow into an oak tree? The caterpillar into a butterfly? What is the intelligence that grows an embryo into a baby? How are the same constellations found in the solar system also found in our own bodies' cellular structures? Life is incomprehensible. Bigger than us.

I don't know what thought is made of, where it comes from and how it works. But I know it does work for us all. There is so much we have yet to discover, which is exciting. Embracing the unknown is where we come alive and activate our genius.

We have this infinitely resilient and creative capacity within us, no matter what, where, how, when or who we are. We are using this precious resource all the time, blessed to be another part of the intelligent fabric of the universe. We are finally free to be and to wonder, secure that we have everything we need.

Aligned with the constant breathing and evolving world we live in, we naturally and effortlessly create the new.

12.
CREATING OUR NEXT STEPS

He who dares wins.

Del Boy

When I stumbled upon the fundamental principles behind our experience, I found the solution to all my problems. I am no longer afraid of my experience. Life had not looked simple and I struggled with my ability to handle it. I now know my uncomfortable and bad feelings are no longer more evidence of my incompetence and shameful inadequacies. I KNOW I am not the problem. And neither are you.

Life becomes an invitation and the world becomes abundant.

Instead of exhausting ourselves with insecure, imaginary scenarios and fearful ways of thinking, there is now opportunity. As a human being, we have been blessed with incredible and unlimited creativity. This realisation creates effortless confidence. Instead of being afraid we know we are able.

Happily, our psychological system is the perfect inner compass to navigate life, always orienting us back to the

Page for Reflection

reliable sun beneath. We can understand and even predict the temporary weather of our feelings. We have found a true and beautiful north star in our experience, a secure and infinite source within us, always there to guide us back home.

Together, we have explored a lot of ideas and information, but it will only help us when we see something true for ourselves. At the beginning of this book, I asked you to jot down a miracle. Take a wee minute to go back and reflect. How does that miracle look today? Has there been any movement? What are you noticing?

If you still feel your miracle is beyond you, I invite you to stay curious. What is it you want when you ask for this miracle? What is it that you think you need?

Why? What is lacking for you?

If there is any work to be done in our lives, this is the work. These questions can illuminate the ideas we have about life. What do we imagine needs to change?

Often what we don't know is more important than what we know. If you still feel entangled, confused and your dreams seem impossible to achieve—it's ok. You are ok. Choose to stay with this hope. Nothing needs to change. What is true for you, me and every living and breathing human is an infinite capacity to create the impossible. The fountain of life provides for us, even if we don't yet see how. Or are too busy to notice it.

Look around you. We have conceived the most astonishing world for ourselves. The screens, pens, desk, ornaments, lamp, chair, clothes, shoes, flooring, doorway, window, plant pot, house, street, town and even the country we are in all started as a simple thought from a curious human mind at some point in time. They had a little idea and set about creating this thing we see before us. From the formless ideas in their minds into the physical forms we now behold.

Indeed the lights are on; the water is running, the electrics are flowing. Look at all those stunning buildings and structures we have created. Bridges that span vast ravines, satellites in space, music we sway to, special effects in movies so good it's hard to believe they are not real. Fellow humans create the seemingly impossible from a simple spark of curiosity and wonder. **This is who we are.**

We are all these amazing creative beings, creating in every moment of our lives and making it up as we go. And I am not just talking about famous creators either. Our route home, the meal at dinnertime, a cup of tea, a clean room, clean hands, a glass of water. We conceive an idea from the unknown, create it in our minds and then bring it into physical being. Then we do it again.

So, what's the game?

Hopefully, understanding that you have everything you need will take a lot off your plate. Now you are free, what would you like to do?

Seeing as you are creating your reality all day, every day. Why not get conscious and choose to live your dreams? Jot down some ideas. Get curious and explore what feels like an inspiring and exciting game you would like to play?

I'm not saying give up your day job just yet, but would you like to learn something new? Take a course. If feeling bad and being scared became more optional? What twinkles your eyes?

Even if you don't have a clue what to do, that's not a problem. No need to get busy, we can just choose to do something that simply feels twinkly today.

No matter what we are up to, we never need to struggle with what we are doing. Whether it be creating a cake, party, painting, home, family, career, part for an engine, plastic stuff, spreadsheets, music, clean streets or a nice cup of coffee. It is possible to do what we would like and have fun doing it.

If you want to play and have some fun, it's no good standing on the sidelines watching or criticising. You are gonna have to jump in and start. Take that first vital and tentative step into the unknown and make each move as the game unfolds. Yes, we might fail and yet equally, we might win!

So nice to win, but what is winning? What is failing? *What if I look stupid / what if no one likes it / what if I fail?* What have we made it mean? What are we afraid of?

Because winning looks like simply enjoying the game, going all in and giving it our best shot. Yes, it may feel difficult, scary or even maddening; but knowing it is a game does indeed change the game. We can play—you know—play? Win or lose, we are already winning because playing IS the fun bit!

Children already know this; we just need to stop pointing them away from it. We are natural learners, born to play and explore, using our innate creativity and magical imagination. The best education keeps that curious and creative flame alive within us.

I will never forget teaching a bunch of 14-year-olds about their extraordinary minds. A boy who kept getting kicked out by the teacher sidled up after class to get his report card filled out. "I'm not thick, am I?" He asked. No gorgeous boy, you are not thick. You are amazing.

Please don't get me wrong; we educate ourselves because learning about life is what generates new connections and ideas. This is how we evolve. We practice and train every day to enjoy presence when we implement our craft effortlessly.

Our minds are not filled with *shoulds* and techniques. Our minds are free; there is lightness and grace. Again we are not thinking about playing—we are playing.

One of my sons forgot how to play football when it all looked serious, when it was all on him. He felt pressured and lost the magic. He stopped taking chances and daring to go for it. He got easily frustrated and angry. Red flags, right? When he became less serious about the outcome and what he had made it mean, he was back to freely playing a game and having fun. Daring to dare and willing to fail.

> Start by doing what's necessary; then do what's possible; and suddenly, you are doing the impossible.
>
> Francis of Assisi

I discussed this idea with my talented friend Claire, a brilliant painter. When she exhibits, people often marvel at how she has created this wonderful painting. She explains that she starts with a simple idea in her head and then makes one simple but bold mark on the blank canvas. Then another. And after thousands of strokes—some fabulous, some not so much—she has created her picture.

Life is a series of possible metaphorical strokes. If we don't like one, we get to create a new one, painting over strokes that haven't worked so well. This is the creative flow, just doing the next right thing.

I know that making that first mark or getting something moving is way harder than keeping it moving. To get into our creative flow, we just need to make that initial step very simple. It can be a teeny little nudge. This is how anything brave, bold and brilliant gets done.

The first step is not to become *a YouTube star.* That is the name of the game. But playing the game begins with opening the app. Then, maybe we could create an account. Perhaps watch a video about how someone else did it? Next, you could play with your camera to make a video you can delete.

You get the picture. The point is just to start playing and stop overthinking. Start where you are and break it down into small, doable tasks. Do one more thing today than yesterday. One stroke, one simple move at a time. There is no right or perfect way, but there is always a way. We simply need to start moving.

Back to our phone analogy. We can open our internal maps application, no matter where we are on our journey, and plug in the destination. The electrical energy within us will then chart a couple of routes. We choose one and off we go, taking each next step and turn. If we go off track, it perfectly calculates our new journey based on wherever we are, in real-time as we travel. It just neutrally recalibrates.

But we can't use this remarkable bit of kit within us if we haven't figured out where we would like to go next. What is a fun sounding destination for you? What will you create next?

Crazy times need our beautiful creative minds

The world may feel chaotic, crazy and extremely serious. But hopefully, the ball will keep on spinning. Each new day will come and go. It's simple; if we don't appreciate how wonderfully ok we are, we will struggle to enjoy a life we love. We will leave feeling good about ourselves and life in the imaginary future.

We'll be alright and feel good when... we get the job / are paid more / sleep better / stop arguing with our partner / have good abs / lose a stone / get an apology / the world feels normal again...

And of course, that day when we finally have it all sorted NEVER. EVER. COMES. Because we have made feeling good about life and ourselves conditional, then we live in a reality where we are never actually being alright and content unless all our conditions are met today.

So no, the diet does not start tomorrow. Getting out of the house, the new project, starting a business, exercising, having more fun, being kinder, enjoying better relationships—can only ever get done in this moment. In our next precious step. The only place we live the dream, or not.

We never need to do more than the next right thing. We can be confident that life is behind us, that it has our back. The only thing that gets in the way of us doing what we love is our ideas about what needs to happen tomorrow or should have happened yesterday.

Our minds may ruminate about the past, but we cannot change it. All we can do is accept that we did our best with what we thought at the time. When we suffer or struggle with the past, we are only ever doing that now, in the present. This moment is the eternal gift where we can step out from our past into the endless possibilities of the future.

But we cannot predict the endless possibilities of the future either. There are too many variables to account for. This is how we get overwhelmed. We become paralysed by trying to imagine and work out all the things that may or may not happen and then make the right choice. We are afraid of all the ways it can go wrong and we may get it wrong. This is worry and anxiety. We catastrophise the future and become completely panicked. We don't need to do that.

Hold on, can it really be that simple? Yes it really can. For as long as we have the gift of life and presence, we are good to go. Tomorrow and yesterday don't exist anywhere else but in our minds, as a succession of new nows we so effortlessly create. We can contemplate the future and the past, we can go wherever our mind takes us, but our helpful psychological system will awaken us when we try to live them now. When our own misunderstandings and mistaken beliefs are holding us back in life today.

No matter what new crazy crisis we are up against, we can KNOW that we are perfectly positioned to thrive. There is no end to the wonders we can create from this knowing.

As long as the neutral, infinite and ingenious life force provides health in our body, beats our heart, pumps our lungs and creates energy to live, we have what we need. It's all a miracle. Take a wonderful long breath out. We don't need to struggle anymore. Create space to abundantly breathe life in. Now really is magically new.

Fill yourself up and allow your beautiful presence to shine out of you, like a warm glowing lantern, lighting up the way home for others. I am ok. You are ok. We are ok.

We have found life's eternal spark of hope and love within us. An extraordinary capacity to create powerful positive connections. It's found in everything. It is where we came from and who we are. Together let's choose to live and share the love.

We are too blessed to be stressed.
If you know someone who is struggling please feel free to pass this book on.

DID YOU ENJOY THIS BOOK?

Please help.

If this book has been helpful I would be so grateful if you could take 5 mins to leave a review on the platform from which you purchased.

A review is the most powerful way to help me reach more readers. Honest reviews of my book help others, like you, decide whether it is a good fit for them.

Thank you!

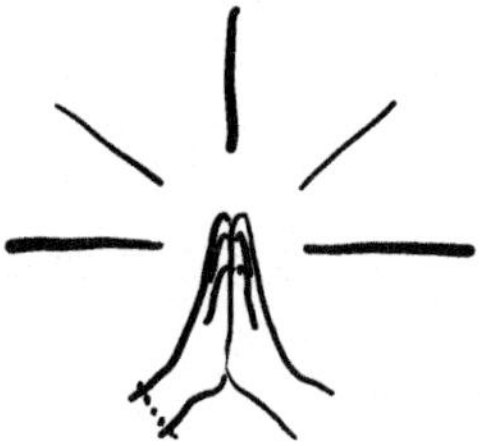

Wise men have come to you to give you of their wisdom. I came to take of your wisdom: and... behold I have found that which is greater than wisdom. It is a flame spirit in you ever gathering more of itself...
You have given me my deeper thirsting after life. Surely there is no greater gift to a man than that which turns all his aims into parching lips and all life into a fountain.

Khalil Gibran

THANK YOU

To my many teachers. No words can express my gratitude for your generosity, inspiration and for, indeed, turning life into a fountain. Through your wisdom this book was born.

I especially want to thank my generous and wonderful mentor Elizabeth Lovius and also the completely zen Ian Watson. Your sense of fun, support and encouragement literally gave me lift off! Thank you to the creative genius of John Scott who helped me back from the deep end to the shallow end where I was free to play again. To Michael Neill, *Creating the Impossible* was the most fun I have had in years and through which I created the epic project *Now is New* - in the most playful way possible :) I have so enjoyed your wisdom and share some of it here.

Thank you to all those involved in founding iheart, (www.iheartprinciples.co.uk) an organisation passionately dedicated to educating our children, but especially the inspirational powerhouses Terry and Brian Rubenstein from whom I have learned so much. Thank you also for all the support from the radiant Debbie Fisher, joyful Dana Arenson, twinkly eyed Stacey Levine and our sorely missed matriarch Shoshanah Kahan. May the organisation impact every child and put us all out of business.

To the clarity and understanding of Sydney Banks and all those who carefully kept the flame of understanding alive. Dr Bill Pettit, Dicken and Coizie Bettinger, George and Linda Pransky, Joe Bailey, Elsie Spittle, Keith Blevens and Valda Monroe, Tzvi Werther, Annette Stein and Jacquie Moses. I am so inspired and grateful for all you do.

You get what you need when you need it. I sure did and could not have written this book without the wise, calm and gentle energy of my amazing editor Emanuel Besorai. Thank you for being the yin to my yang.

I want to thank from the bottom of my heart all those that gave their time and energy to read the manuscript at various stages. Your feedback has been invaluable: Nima Tayebi, Nick Jaffee, Alex Halliday, Christine Friend, Juliet Carter, Debra Berzin-Cohen, Freda Lawlor and Rosa Matthews—your kind words of encouragement kept me going. Also Lizzie Edwards, Marcia O'Regan, Jo Oli, Kriss Fasunloye and Dyliss Faife for the love and keeping me on track. To Maya Patrick for being a beautiful gem of inspiration and the sparkly Rachel Patrick for being a rock star and sounding board in this project. Exciting things to come! Thomas Brosnan, genuinely thank you for your support and encouragement. And Chrissy Kelly. Together we are indeed creating the next steps to helping one million young people, especially those that struggle. Just so much love and appreciation to all my friends and family for your support.

I want to give a shout out to the staff at Costa and Gails, good coffee, good vibes and where this book was written!

Naz, I could not have done it without you, your clarity, care and daily dose of common sense. Nic, you have lived and shared the love since day one. My mum Lisa—I miss you. Jim and Pat—thank you for all your love and encouragement in this endeavour and the rest! And a special thanks for the most practical support Mike. The hot dinners and smoothies after being in Costa writing away all day were the best. And finally, thank you to my greatest teachers and best friends Rafael, Canon, Sol and Aïda. Pure love and gratitude you are by my side.

ABOUT THE AUTHOR

Katherine Chidiac is a mum, creative, entrepreneur and facilitator. She lives in North London with her family and little old lady pup, Lulu.

Kat tends to do whatever she loves, whenever possible—spending most of her 'working hours' trying to create cool new stuff or connecting with amazing people. She can also be found hanging out with her kids, watching footie (her sons / beloved Arsenal), listening to people talk for hours on YouTube, playing cards, dancing, singing in the car (or even better, a karaoke booth), cooking, doing the dishes, drinking tea and taking a nice hot bath at the end of a long day.

Kat founded the campaign Now is New in 2021 to reach one million young people and help them create a life they love. It's pretty simple folks—when we feel ok, we do ok...

For updates, continued support, or if you would like to connect, the project is found across social channels
@_nowisnew Insta / TikTok / YouTube
Plus, look out for our free new app—coming soon!

For further resources and courses, please visit
www.nowisnew.co.uk

Printed in Great Britain
by Amazon

81781990R00088